Pediatric Anesthesia

Pediatric Anesthesia

A Quick Pocket Reference

Second Edition

Edmond C. Bloch, M.B., Ch.B., FRCA, FRCS(I)
Associate Professor Emeritus of Anesthesia and Former Director of Pediatric Anesthesia, Duke University Medical Center, Durham, North Carolina

Brian Ginsberg, M.B, Ch.B., FFA(SA)
Associate Professor of Anesthesia and Director of Acute Pain Services, Duke University Medical Center, Durham, North Carolina

Foreword by

Merel H. Harmel, M.D.
Professor and Chairman Emeritus of Anesthesiology, Duke University Medical Center, Durham, North Carolina

BUTTERWORTH HEINEMANN

Boston Oxford Auckland Johannesburg Melbourne New Delhi

Every effort has been made to ensure that the drug dosage schedules within this text are accurate and conform to standards accepted at time of publication. However, as treatment recommendations vary in the light of continuing research and clinical experience, the reader is advised to verify drug dosage schedules herein with information found on product information sheets. This is especially true in cases of new or infrequently used drugs.

Recognizing the importance of preserving what has been written, Butterworth–Heinemann prints its books on acid-free paper whenever possible.

Butterworth–Heinemann supports the efforts of American Forests and the Global ReLeaf program in its campaign for the betterment of trees, forests, and our environment.

Library of Congress Cataloging-in-Publication Data
Bloch, Edmond C.
Pediatric anesthesia : a quick pocket reference / Edmond C. Bloch, Brian Ginsberg ; foreword by Merel H. Harmel. -- 2nd ed.
p. cm.
Includes bibliographical references and index.
ISBN 0-7506-7142-4
1. Pediatric anesthesia Handbooks, manuals, etc. I. Ginsberg, Brian. II. Title.
[DNLM: 1. Anesthesia--Infant Handbooks. 2. Anesthesia--Child Handbooks. WO 231 B651p 1999]
RD139.B56 1999
617.9'6798--dc21
DNLM/DLC
for Library of Congress 99-19066
CIP

British Library Cataloguing-in-Publication Data
A catalogue record for this book is available from the British Library.

The publisher offers special discounts on bulk orders of this book.
For information, please contact:

Manager of Special Sales
Butterworth–Heinemann
225 Wildwood Avenue
Woburn, MA 01801-2041
Tel: 781-904-2500
Fax: 781-904-2620

For information on all Butterworth–Heinemann publications available, contact our World Wide Web home page at: http://www.bh.com

10 9 8 7 6 5 4 3 2 1

Printed in the United States of America

Contents

Foreword

I have known Edmond Bloch since he came to the United States from South Africa in 1977. Although fully trained, he had to enter a residency program to qualify for licensure in the United States. He was readily accepted into the program at Duke, where I was chair. His practice in South Africa was that of a generalist, but it became apparent that he had a love for—and special skill in—pediatric anesthesia. This undoubtedly can be traced to his association with an outstanding mentor, Jackson Rees, the eminent pediatric anesthetist in Liverpool. His interest and superb clinical skill in pediatric anesthesia added immeasurably to the educational and clinical goals of our department, resulting in his appointment as Chief of the Pediatric Anesthesia Program at Duke, a post he filled with distinction.

Dr. Bloch soon recognized the need for providing up-to-the-minute data, together with a precise outline of procedures that could be readily accessed by students, residents, and faculty from other specialty areas (whose familiarity with pediatric anesthesia may not have been current). It became clear that his notes, which he made available to all those on the service, might be useful for a wider audience. Thus, in 1994 was born the first edition of *Pediatric Anesthesia: A Pocket Companion*—a small, distinctive volume that easily fit into a pocket. Indeed, this small compendium has found a useful place in the day-to-day armamentarium of students, residents, nurse anesthetists, and practitioners within and without the operating theater. It is valued especially for its concise, precise, and easily obtainable information. To have a formulary and information about standard procedures at one's fingertips is particularly useful for those beginning their training in pediatric anesthesia and for those whose daily encounters in pediatric anesthesia are limited.

The success of the first edition has warranted a second edition. In the intervening 5 years, the anesthesiologist's involvement in the management of pain in infants and children has increased significantly. In addition, the participation of the pediatric anesthesiologist in off-site procedures has been extended. Furthermore, the opportunity to update the formulary, dosages, procedures, and their presentation has been appropriately amplified in keeping with the objectives of a pocket reference. Brian Ginsberg has joined Dr. Bloch in authoring this edition, and his expertise in pain management and off-site anesthesia has significantly added to the book's value.

In its revised and extended format, *Pediatric Anesthesia: A Quick Pocket Reference* will continue to occupy a unique niche and admirably serve the needs of pediatric anesthesia training and practice.

Merel H. Harmel

Preface

The days when a bottle of ether and a mask met the anesthesia provider's needs ended long ago (although ether is still a valuable and safe tool in many underdeveloped areas). The scope and complexity of information related to our specialty and its many subdivisions has increased enormously; it is difficult, if not impossible, for one person to be familiar with it all. The purpose of this book is to provide readily available information for those attending to patients in the perioperative period. We hope that it will serve all anesthesia providers, from residents to veterans.

The material is presented in an organized fashion, with an extensive index for ready access. Some material from the first edition has been preserved, but it has been reorganized and updated. As much as possible, we have avoided repetition. A list of recommended texts provides a resource for further reading. Blank pages are provided for those who wish to add notes in the light of their experiences. It has been kept to a convenient pocket size for easy availability.

To ensure that the information provided is accurate and conforms to standards accepted at the time of publication, the content has been checked with multiple sources. Drug dosages have received particular attention. However, because patient needs and treatment recommendations vary, and in view of the possibility of human error or changes in medical science, it is the responsibility of the individual physician to determine dosages and treatment for each patient. The reader is thus advised to verify drug dosage schedules herein with information found on product information sheets, in the references provided, or in standard texts. This is especially true in cases of new or infrequently used drugs.

In this book, *neonate* refers to the first month of life; *infant* to the first year of life; and *child* to the years thereafter, until the age of 12. *Adolescence* is considered to be the period between the ages of 13 and 19 years. Although IM doses are provided, we prefer the IV route whenever possible, because it is painless and the response is more predictable.

EB
BG

Suggestions for Further Reading

PEDIATRICS

Behrman RE, Kliegman RM (eds). Nelson Essentials of Pediatrics (3rd ed). Philadelphia: WB Saunders, 1998.

DISEASES OF THE NEWBORN

Taeusch HW, Ballard RA (eds). Avery's Diseases of the Newborn (7th ed). Philadelphia: WB Saunders, 1998.

PEDIATRIC LIFE SUPPORT (CPR), BASIC AND ADVANCED

Chameides L, Hazinski MF (eds). Pediatric Advanced Life Support. Subcommittee on Pediatric Resuscitation. Dallas: American Heart Association, 1997.

PEDIATRIC ANESTHESIA

Gregory GA (ed). Pediatric Anesthesia (3rd ed). New York: Churchill Livingstone, 1994.

Motoyama EK, Davis PJ (eds). Smith's Anesthesia for Infants and Children (6th ed). St. Louis: Mosby–Year Book, 1996.

REGIONAL ANESTHESIA

Committee on Drugs of the American Academy of Pediatrics. Guidelines for monitoring and management of pediatric patients during and after sedation for diagnostic and therapeutic procedures. Pediatrics 1992;89: 1110–1115.

Dalens B (ed). Regional Anesthesia in Infants, Children and Adolescents. London: Williams & Wilkins Waverly Europe, 1995.

Downey DA, Doyle E. Epidural and subarachnoid blockade in children. Anaesthesia 1998;53:980–1001. (*Editors' note: An excellent review article.*)

PEDIATRIC CARDIAC ANESTHESIA

Lake CL (ed). Pediatric Cardiac Anesthesia (3rd ed). Stamford, CT: Appleton & Lange, 1997.

PEDIATRIC AIRWAY

Riazi J. The Difficult Pediatric Airway. In JL Beumof (ed), Airway Management: Principles and Practice. St. Louis: Mosby–Year Book, 1996.

PEDIATRIC PAIN

Ashburn MA, Rice LJ (eds). The Management of Pain. New York: Churchill Livingstone, 1997. (*Editors' note: See Chapter 39, The Management of Acute Pain in the Child, and Chapter 40, The Management of Procedure-Related Pain in the Child.*)

Bell C, Kain ZN (eds). The Pediatric Anesthesia Handbook (2nd ed). St. Louis: Mosby–Year Book, 1996.

Deshpande JK, Tobias JD (eds). The Pediatric Pain Handbook. St. Louis: Mosby–Year Book, 1996.

Zideman DA. Pediatric and neonatal life support. Br J Anaesth 1997;79:181.

Abbreviations

ACE	angiotensin-converting enzyme
ACT	activated clotting time
CNS	central nervous system
CSF	cerebrospinal fluid
CT	computed tomography
D5W	a solution of 5% dextrose in water
DDAVP	1-desamino-8-D-arginine vasopressin
ECG	electrocardiography
EMG	electromyography
ET	endotracheal; intratracheally
GI	gastrointestinal
Hb	hemoglobin
HIV	human immunodeficiency virus
HTLV	human T-cell lymphoma virus
IM	intramuscular
IO	intraosseous
IV	intravenous
MAC	mean alveolar concentration
MRI	magnetic resonance imaging
NPO	nothing by mouth
P_{50}	partial pressure of O_2 of whole blood at 50% SaO_2
PaO_2	partial pressure of O_2 in arterial blood
P_{ECO_2}	partial pressure of CO_2 in expired gas
P_{ETCO_2}	partial pressure of end-tidal CO_2
PO	oral
PR	per rectum

prn	as the need arises
PTC	post-tetanic count
Sao_2	saturation of arterial blood with oxygen
SQ	subcutaneous
THAM	tromethamine
TOF	train-of-four

1

Preoperative Considerations

GOALS

- Minimize apprehension and any untoward effects of surgery and anesthesia (e.g., pain, nausea, emesis).
- Provide sedation with amnesia and, if necessary, analgesia. Allowing a parent or other responsible adult to be present (when appropriate) until the patient loses consciousness can be extremely helpful during induction.
- Provide supplementation of anesthesia.

INCUBATION PERIOD OF CHILDHOOD DISEASES

Diphtheria	3 days (range, 1–7 days)
Meningococcal infection	Up to 1 wk
Mumps	17 days (range, 14–24 days)
Rubella (German measles)	14–21 days
Rubeola (measles)	10 days (range, 7–18 days)
Scarlet fever	2–3 days
Tetanus	5–14 days, but may be months
Varicella (chickenpox)	16 days (range, 10–20 days)
Variola (smallpox)	12 days (range, 12–16 days)

AMERICAN SOCIETY OF ANESTHESIOLOGISTS' CLASSIFICATION OF PHYSICAL STATUS

Class 1	Normal healthy patient
Class 2	Patient with mild systemic disease
Class 3	Patient with severe systemic disease that limits activity but is not incapacitating
Class 4	Patient with incapacitating systemic disease that is a constant threat to life
Class 5	Moribund patient who is not expected to survive for 24 hrs with or without operation
E	Emergency

PREOPERATIVE FEEDING RESTRICTIONS[331]

Patients 6 Months Old and Younger

- Normal feeding until 4 hrs before anesthesia
- For next 2 hrs, water, breast milk, or clear apple juice only
- For 2 hrs before anesthesia, NPO

Patients 7 Months to 3 Years Old

- Clear fluids only, commencing 6 hrs before anesthesia
- Clear fluids stopped 2–3 hrs before anesthesia

Patients Older Than 3 Years

- Clear fluids only, commencing 8 hrs before anesthesia
- Clear fluids stopped 2–3 hrs before anesthesia

Patients at risk (e.g., those with gastroesophageal reflux or requiring emergency surgery) must receive special consideration.

DRUGS FOR PREOPERATIVE MEDICATION

Atropine	0.02 mg/kg IM and PO[119]; 0.01 mg/kg IV.
	Minimum single dose: 0.1 mg/kg.
Captopril[247]	0.3 mg/kg PO 1.5 hrs preoperatively to facilitate controlled hypertension.
	Infants: half this dose.
Chloral hydrate	<77 mg/kg PO[37] and PR.
	Neonates: <50 mg/kg.
	No analgesic properties.
Chlorpromazine[247]	0.5 mg/kg IM and IV; 1.0 mg/kg PO.
Cimetidine	5–10 mg/kg IV and PO.[324]
Clonidine	4.0 µg/kg PO 1.5 hrs preoperatively; slow onset (±1.5 hrs).[207,224]
	2.5 µg/kg PR 20 mins before induction.[213,225]
Diazepam[33]	0.1–0.3 mg/kg IV; onset in 3–4 mins.
	0.1–0.2 mg/kg PO; onset in 30–60 mins.
	0.75 mg/kg PR; 0.3–0.4 mg/kg IM.
Diphenhydramine	1.0 mg/kg IV, IM, and PO.
	Neonates: half this dose.
Droperidol	As sedative: 0.15 mg/kg IM; 0.08–0.16 mg/kg IV[308]; 0.2 mg/kg PO.

	As antiemetic premedication: 75 μg/kg IV and PO.[40]
Famotidine	0.15 mg/kg[123] to 0.5 mg/kg PO.
Fentanyl	0.5–1.0 μg/kg IV; may be repeated q5min to a maximum of 4–5 μg/kg. Watch respiration. Half-life: 2.0–3.5 hrs.
Fentanyl lozenge	Oral transmucosal fentanyl citrate (Oralet). 10 μg/kg by oral transmucosal route 30 mins before procedure.[128,223,247,302] Peak effect in 20–30 mins; duration: 30–60 mins.[382] Depression of ventilation lasts longer than analgesia.[382] Respiration must be monitored after administration.[131] Contraindicated in patients younger than 2 yrs or weighing ≤15 kg.
Glycopyrrolate	10 μg/kg IM or IV; 20 μg/kg PO.
Hydroxyzine	0.6 mg/kg PO.
Ketamine[121,256]	2–5 mg/kg IM; 0.5–1.0 mg/kg IV; 8–10 mg/kg PR. 6–10 mg/kg PO; onset of sedation: 10–20 mins.[299] Nasally: 6 mg/kg 30 mins before procedure.[227]
Meperidine	1.0–1.5 mg/kg IV or IM.[259]

	1.0–2.0 mg/kg PO; maximum dose, 100 mg/kg.[389] Half-life: 2–3 hrs.[347] Newborn: 0.5 mg/kg/dose IV or IM; 0.5–1.0 mg/kg/dose PO.[163] Monitor for respiratory depression, which is reversible with naloxone.
Metoclopramide	0.15 mg/kg IM; 0.15 mg/kg IV[118]; 0.2 mg/kg PO. May be used IV after induction and again in the postoperative period. Onset in 1–3 mins; duration: 1.5–3.0 hrs.
Midazolam	0.75 mg/kg PO for age 1–6 yrs and 0.4 for age 6–12 yrs.[32,34,101] 0.08–0.30 mg/kg IM. Incremental doses of 0.1 mg/kg IV; titrated to effect[312]; maximum, 0.7 mg/kg. Jet injection: 0.10–0.15 mg/kg.[324] Nasally: 0.2–0.3 mg/kg[256]; stings and tastes unpleasant; onset in 10 mins, peaks in 15 mins.[345] 0.5–1.0 mg/kg PR.[51,256] Sublingual: 0.2 mg/kg for 0.5- to 10-year-olds.[298] Neonate: IV or IM for sedation,[163] 0.07–0.20 mg/kg/dose. Good oral sedative for minor procedures (e.g., IV line).

Morphine sulfate	100–200 μg/kg IM and IV; 200–500 μg/kg PO.[247] Neonate: 50–100 μg/kg/dose IV, IM, or SQ.[163] Monitor respiratory rate and SaO_2. Half-life: 3.9 hrs in children; 6.8 hrs in first week of life.[100]
Ondansetron	150 μg/kg IV.[130] 0.1 mg/kg PO rounded to the nearest 2 mg.[168]
Pentazocine	1.5 mg/kg IM.
Pentobarbital[259]	For premedication: 3–4 mg/kg PO. For sedation: 4 mg/kg IV q2min to the desired result, with maximum dose of 10 mg/kg.
Phenobarbital[257]	1–3 mg/kg PO, IM, or IV, 1.0–1.5 hrs preoperatively.
Promethazine	0.5–1.0 mg/kg IM; 0.25–0.50 mg/kg IV; 0.5–1.0 mg/kg PO.
Ranitidine[84]	0.25–1.00 mg/kg IV[182]; 2.0 mg/kg PO
Scopolamine[2,379]	0.01 mg/kg IM (minimum dose of 0.1 mg/kg, maximum dose of 0.4 mg/kg). Stronger salivary suppression and more sedative effect than atropine. Reversible with physostigmine, 0.035 mg/kg IM or slow IV.
Sufentanil[362]	Nasally: 1.5–4.4 mg/kg.
Tropisetron[369]	0.1 mg/kg IV.

ORAL PREMEDICATION FOR PEDIATRIC OUTPATIENTS

The following combination can be used to decrease preoperative problems without prolonging recovery[38]:

Diazepam: 0.2 mg/kg
Meperidine: 1.5 mg/kg
Atropine: 0.02 mg/kg

SEDATION

Conscious Sedation

Conscious sedation is a medically controlled state of depressed consciousness that has the following requirements:

Informed written parental consent
Preoperative feeding restrictions as for any anesthetic
Uninterrupted observation of the patient and monitoring of the following conditions:

- Independent maintenance of a patent airway and respiration
- Maintenance of protective reflexes
- Maintenance of responsiveness to verbal commands
- Continuous pulse oximetry and heart rate
- Intermittent blood pressure

The anesthesia provider should be aware that loss of consciousness, though unlikely, may occur.

Equipment for Conscious Sedation

- Airway management kit containing, for example, laryngoscopes, tracheal tubes, oral airways, and masks, including laryngeal airways.
- Oxygen delivery system capable of delivering 100% O_2 for 1 hr.
- ECG and pulse oximeter for monitoring Sao_2.
- Noninvasive blood pressure apparatus.
- Functional O_2 cylinder, or a wall supply.
- Cart with all emergency requirements (appropriate drugs for resuscitation are detailed in Chapter 15) and equipment to provide or supplement ventilation (self-inflating bag).
- Suction source and suction catheters.
- Equipment and drugs to be regularly checked by an established schedule.
- Provision for safe patient transport.

Deep Sedation

Deep sedation is a medically controlled state of depressed consciousness or unconsciousness from which the patient is not easily aroused. It can involve loss of protective reflexes, the inability to maintain a patent airway, and the absence of response to verbal or physical stimulation. Deep sedation approaches the state of general anesthesia. Requirements for deep sedation are the same as those described for conscious sedation, but an ECG monitor should also be used, and a defibrillator suitable for pediatric patients must be available. The use of a precordial stethoscope and capnograph is strongly advised.[335]

ANESTHESIA IN A REMOTE LOCATION

Some procedures are performed outside the operating room or at remote locations. Such procedures include radiation therapy, radiologic imaging, bone marrow transplants, and MRI. The requirements described for conscious or deep sedation in these locations are the same as those appropriate for general anesthesia.

SUGGESTED MEDICATION REGIMENS FOR SEDATION WITH OR WITHOUT ANALGESIA

- Chloral hydrate[203]: for sedation, 15–25 mg/kg/dose PO or PR; as a hypnotic, 50–100 mg/kg/dose.[345] Maximum: 2 g/dose. Does not provide analgesia.
- Pentobarbital: 2–6 mg/kg IV. Infuse slowly in increments of 0.25–0.50 of the total calculated dose, titrating against the patient's response.[17,99] A very good sedative—useful for CT scans. Does not provide analgesia.
- Methohexital 5%: 10 mg/km IM[18]; 25 mg/kg of a 10% solution PR.[205] Most useful for sedation PR. No analgesia. Watch for respiratory depression.
- Midazolam: 0.50–0.75 mg/kg PO for sedation during MRI.[111]
    IV: incremental doses of 0.1 mg/kg, titrated to effect. Maximum: 0.7 mg/kg.

PR: 0.3–0.7 mg/kg. Onset 10–15 mins; duration: 2.5 hrs.[345]

IM: 0.1–0.3 mg/kg. However, 0.08 mg/kg has been found to provide good sedation. Onset: 10–15 mins; duration: 2.5 hrs.[345,346]

Nasally: 0.2–0.4 mg/kg. Onset: 10 mins; peak: 15 mins; duration: 1 hr.[345] Stings and the taste is unpleasant.

Neonate: 0.07–0.20 mg/kg/dose IV or IM for sedation.[163]

- Propofol: If patient does not have an IV in situ, induce with sevoflurane/N_2O or halothane/N_2O and insert an IV cannula.[129] Then give 1.0–2.0 mg/kg IV as a loading dose and *start* an infusion at 100 μg/kg/min; titrate to required effect. Inhalational agents may then be discontinued.
- Ketamine: 0.5–1.0 mg/kg IV repeated to effect. Short acting (15 mins if only one dose has been given).[344] Atropine controls salivation. Conscious sedation cannot be achieved with ketamine. Ketamine provides excellent analgesia and is very good for short painful procedures. Be aware of the possibility of postoperative dysphoria, which is more common in older children. IM ketamine at a dose of 3 mg/kg is most useful for sedating an otherwise uncontrollable child before, for instance, an IV insertion.[344]
- Sufentanil is not recommended for conscious sedation.[345]
- So-called lytic cocktails (DPT [Demerol, meperidine, chlorpromazine] and APT [atropine, meperidine, promethazine]) should never be used.[206]

Monitor the patient continuously after the procedure until the patient is alert. Pulse oximetry (SaO_2) is especially important.

Some Drugs Used for Sedation before Procedures

Drug	*Route*	*Dose*	*Peak effect*	*Duration*
Anxiolytics/sedatives				
Diazepam	PO	0.1–0.5 mg/kg	30–60 mins	6–20 hrs
	IV	0.1–0.3 mg/kg	3–4 mins	Dose dependent (>2 hrs)
	PR	0.2–0.3 mg/kg	40–60 mins	6–20 hrs
Midazolam	PO	0.50–0.75 mg/kg (max: <5 mg/kg)	10–30 mins	60 mins
	Sublingual	0.2–0.4 mg/kg	10–15 mins	60 mins
	IV	0.05–0.15 mg/kg	3–4 mins	Dose dependent
	PR	0.5–1.0 mg/kg	5–20 mins	60 mins
Chloral hydrate				
as hypnotic	PO or PR	50–75 mg/kg (max: 1g)	20–40 mins	6–8 hrs
as sedative	PO or PR	15–25 mg/kg	20–40 mins	6–8 hrs
Opioids				
Fentanyl	Sublingual (oral transmucosal fentanyl citrate [Oralet])	5–10 μg/kg	10–15 mins	1–2 hrs
	IV	0.5–1.0 mg/kg	1–3 mins	30–40 mins
Morphine	PO	0.2–0.5 mg/kg	60–90 mins	2–4 hrs
	IM	0.1–0.2 mg/kg	15–30 mins	2–4 hrs
	IV	0.03–0.05 mg/kg	5–10 mins	2–4 hrs
Meperidine	PO	1–2 mg/kg	60–90 mins	2–4 hrs
	IV	0.5–1.0 mg/kg	2–4 mins	2–4 hrs

continued

Drug	Route	Dose	Peak effect	Duration
Anesthetic agents				
Ketamine	PO	5–6 mg/kg	20–30 mins	0.5–1.0 hr
	IM	2–5 mg/kg	1–3 mins	0.5–2.0 hrs
	Nasally	3 mg/kg	10 mins	0.5–1.0 hr
	IV	1–2 mg/kg	0.5–2.0 mins	0.5–1.0 hr
Methohexital	PR	20–30 mg/kg	6–10 mins	2–4 hrs
	IM	10 mg/kg	4–10 mins	2–4 hrs
Propofol	IV	0.5–3.0 mg/kg	30–60 secs	5–10 mins

ASPIRATION PROPHYLAXIS[90,253]

Metoclopramide	0.15 mg/kg IV
Cimetidine	7.5 mg/kg PO[247]
Ranitidine	2 mg/kg PO[89]
Sodium citrate	0.5 mL/kg PO (0.3 molar)

NAUSEA AND VOMITING PROPHYLAXIS

- Droperidol: ≤75 μg/kg IV; best given at induction.[39,40] Watch for side effects.
- Diphenhydramine: For routine use, 50–100 μg/kg IV after induction.[229] For strabismus surgery, 0.5 mg/kg PO preoperatively is markedly effective.[289]
- Granisetron: Used mostly for chemotherapy-induced nausea and vomiting. Recommended dose is 10 μg/kg IV 30 mins before initiation of therapy,[384] but in one study, 40 μg/kg IV was used successfully in children for strabismus surgery.[310] No pediatric oral dose is available. Its safety and efficacy in children 2 yrs old or younger has not been demonstrated.

- Lorazepam: 10 μg/kg IV. Best given at induction.[137]
- Ondansetron: 150 μg/kg IV after induction.[130]
- Propofol: 2.5–3.0 mg/kg IV for induction; has good antiemetic properties.[181] Use approximately half this dose if patient is well sedated with opiates or if younger than 2 wks. Pain on injection may be reduced by adding lidocaine, 0.2 mg/kg, and injecting into a large vein. Small veins on the dorsum of the hand should be avoided if possible; the antecubital fossa is suggested.[325] Follow-up infusion rate is 100–200 μg/kg/min.

ENDOCARDITIS PROPHYLAXIS[320,357]

Cardiac Patients at Risk

Risk factors for cardiac patients include previous bacterial endocarditis, most congenital cardiac malformations, acquired valvular malfunction (e.g., surgery, rheumatic fever), prosthetic valves, mitral valve prolapse with regurgitation, and transvenous pacemakers.

Dental or Surgical Patients at Risk

Risk factors for dental or surgical patients include dental procedures that provoke bleeding, tonsillectomy or adenoidectomy, surgery involving intestinal or respiratory mucosa, gallbladder surgery, cystoscopy, urethral dilatation, bladder catheterization, infected urinary tract surgery, surgery of infected tissue, and shunts (hydrocephalic and dialysis) and fistulas.

Prophylaxis for Dental, Oral, or Upper Respiratory Tract Procedures

The following medications are for patients at risk, including those with prosthetic heart valves:

Oral Medications

- Amoxicillin, 50 mg/kg PO 1 hr preoperatively, then 25 mg/kg 6 hrs later.
- If the patient is allergic to penicillin: erythromycin, 25 mg/kg PO 2 hrs before the procedure, repeated 10 mg/kg PO 6 hrs later. Alternatively: clindamycin, 10 mg/kg PO 1 hr preoperatively, then 15 mg/kg 6 hrs later.

Intravenous Medications

- IM: Ampicillin, 50 mg/kg and gentamicin, 2 mg/kg 30 mins preoperatively.
  IV: Both these antibiotics in the same doses over 30 mins preoperatively.
- If the patient is allergic to penicillin: clindamycin, 10 kg/kg PO 2 hrs preoperatively, then 5 mg/kg 6 hrs later.
- If the patient is allergic to penicillin and at high risk: vancomycin,* 20 mg/kg IV over 60 mins, 1 hr preoperatively.
- No second dose is necessary.

---

*Vancomycin always must be given as a slow IV infusion over 60 mins. Allergic reactions can be severe, especially when the dose is administered too quickly. Diphenhydramine, 1 mg/kg, is the best antihistaminic for this purpose; steroids and circulatory support may be needed.

Prophylaxis for Genitourinary or Gastrointestinal Procedures

- If the patient is at low risk and can take oral medicines: ampicillin, 50 mg/kg PO 1 hr preoperatively, followed by the same dose 6 hrs later.
- If the patient is not at low risk: ampicillin, 50 mg/kg IM and gentamicin, 2 mg/kg IM 30 mins preoperatively; or both these antibiotics IV in the same doses over 30 mins preoperatively. Repeat this dose 8 hrs later.
- If the patient is allergic to penicillin: vancomycin,* 20 mg/kg IV slowly over 1 hr preoperatively, plus gentamicin, 2 mg/kg 30 mins preoperatively. Repeat once 8–12 hrs later.

Special Cases

Rheumatic Fever

Patients on oral penicillin prophylaxis to prevent a recurrence should be given erythromycin, 20 mg/kg PO 2 hrs preoperatively and 10 mg/kg 6 hrs later.

Patients on Anticoagulants

Use PO or IV routes of administration. IM injections are contraindicated.

---

*Vancomycin always must be given as a slow IV infusion over 60 mins. Allergic reactions can be severe, especially when the dose is administered too quickly. Diphenhydramine, 1 mg/kg, is the best antihistaminic for this purpose; steroids and circulatory support may be needed.

ANTINEOPLASTIC AGENTS

- Cyclophosphamide acutely induces cardiomyopathy after a cumulative dose of more than 120 mg/m^2.
- Doxorubicin (Adriamycin [an anthracycline]) also induces cardiomyopathy, the incidence of which increases as the cumulative dose rises. The critical level is reported to be 550 mg/m^2 but may be as low as 100 mg/m^2. Thus, preoperative cardiologic investigation (ECG, chest x-ray, and echocardiography) is recommended[46,61] if the cumulative dose of doxorubicin is more than 250 mg/m^2.

NOTES

NOTES

2

Induction of Anesthesia

RAPID SEQUENCE INDUCTION

Rapid sequence induction is used to prevent gastroesophageal reflux during induction and intubation. After preoxygenation of approximately 2 mins, cricoid pressure (the Sellick maneuver) is applied as the child loses consciousness and is maintained until the trachea is intubated.

Drugs used in rapid sequence induction are as follows:

1. Atropine, 0.02 mg/kg IV
2. Thiopental, 7–8 mg/kg IV in infants; 4–6 mg/kg IV if older than 1 yr, or Propofol, 2–3 mg/kg IV
3. Succinylcholine, 2–3 mg/kg IV, or rocuronium, 1.0–1.2 mg/kg IV

AWAKE INTUBATION

Awake intubation[287] is sometimes used in neonates and infants when induction of general anesthesia is inadvisable until the airway is secured. Ability to visualize the larynx or intubate the trachea may be hampered (e.g., by malformation or obstruction of the upper airway). Awake intubation provokes a marked increase in autonomic responses and intracranial pressure. Atropine, 0.02 mg/kg IV, is followed by preoxygenation for 2 mins before intubation is attempted. Lidocaine, 1.5 mg/kg IV; fentanyl, 1–3 μg/kg IV; or a combination of the two may be used to control noxious stimuli.

INHALATION AGENTS[30,133]

MAC is defined as the end-tidal concentration of a gas or vapor at which 50% of patients move in response to surgical skin incision.[170]

Agent	*Neonates*	*1–6 mos*	*6–12 mos*	*12–24 mos*	*Children*
Desflurane[104]	9.16%	9.42%	9.92%	8.72%	7.89%
Enflurane	—	—	—	1.69%	—
Halothane[28]	0.87%	1.2%	1.98%	0.97%	0.87%
Isoflurane[29]	1.6%	1.87%	1.8%	1.6%	1.6%
N_2O[113] (predicted)	—	—	—	—	109%
Sevoflurane[112,135]	3.2%	3.2%	2.5%	2.5%	2.49%[112]

- MAC values are reduced 22–25% by adding 60% nitrous oxide.[117]
- In a more recent publication, inhalation agent values very similar to those presented here were reported.[300]
- Children tolerate higher doses of epinephrine during halothane anesthesia than adults.[188] The dose of epinephrine should not be >10 μg/kg/20 mins.[187,189] Some have recommended ≤5 μg/kg/10 mins.[86]
- Hypertension and tachycardia are more common than dysrhythmias.

DRUGS

Alfentanil	As the main anesthetic agent: 100 μg/kg IV, followed by an average infusion rate of 2.4 μg/kg/min.[316] As a supplement to N_2O/O_2 general anesthesia: 20–25 μg/kg IV,[126] then an IV infusion of 1–3 μg/kg/min.[122] As adjunct to other agents: 20–25 μg/kg IV.[126] Half-life: 6–12 mins.[347]
Diazepam	0.1–0.2 mg/kg IV.
Droperidol	0.15–0.20 mg/kg IV.[177]
Etomidate	0.2–0.3 mg/kg IV.[248]
Fentanyl	As adjunct to other agents: 1–5 μg/kg IV. As the main anesthetic agent: 50–100 μg/kg IV. For cardiac surgery: ≤150 μg/kg IV. Large doses may require postoperative ventilation. Consider reducing doses for neonates and infants.[126] Half-life: 2.0–3.5 hrs.
Ketamine	2 mg/kg IV; 8–10 mg/kg IM; 15 mg/kg PR. 6 mg/kg PO in a little soda or cherry syrup 0.5 hr preoperatively.[121] Infants younger than 6 mos may need the higher doses.[48] Onset of PO ketamine: 20–30 mins.[121]

	Infusion for sedation: 5–20 μg/kg/min; start at lower dose and titrate as needed.[247] Ketamine is a useful induction agent for infants with cyanotic heart disease (if the infants are normovolemic), because it maintains both systemic and pulmonary vascular resistance.[364]
Meperidine	For premedication: 1.5–3.0 mg/kg PO; or 1 mg/kg IM or IV. Maximum total dose: 100 mg/kg.[389] Half-life: 2–3 hrs.[347] With N_2O in the neonate: 0.5–1.0 mg/kg for cardiac cases.[175]
Methohexital	2 mg/kg IV; 8–10 mg/kg IM; 25 mg/kg PR of a 10% solution. Most useful for induction of sedation by PR route.
Morphine[126]	As adjunct to other agents: 0.05–0.10 mg/kg. As the main anesthetic agent: 1–2 mg/kg. Postoperative ventilation may be needed. Half-life: 3.9 hrs in children; 6.8 hrs in first week of life.[100]
Propofol	IV propofol can be painful. Lidocaine, 0.2 mg/kg IV, administered before or mixed with propofol may minimize the pain. Locating a large vein (e.g., the

antecubital fossa instead of dorsum of the hand) is suggested.[325]

Induction: 3 mg/kg IV; younger children may require more.[118]

Infusion: 1–2 mg/kg initial bolus, then 300 μg/kg/min for 15 mins; reduce to 150 μg/kg/min and titrate as indicated by blood pressure and heart rate.[181]

For MRI: Induce with halothane/N_2O or sevoflurane/N_2O and insert an IV cannula. Give 2 mg/kg propofol IV as a loading dose and start an infusion at 100 μg/kg/min. Titrate to effect. Halothane may then be discontinued.[129]

MRI sedation with laryngeal mask insertion: Induce with 2.5 mg/kg and follow with an infusion of 83 μg/kg/min.[282]

Monitored anesthesia care sedation: Mix propofol, 8 mg, and alfentanil, 0.08 mg, in each mL and start an infusion at 60–80 μg/kg/min. Titrate to patient's requirements.[131]

Propofol is not currently licensed for use in critically ill children in intensive care units.[131] Metabolic acidosis during infusion and neurologic sequelae after withdrawal have been reported in patients with respiratory infections.[283,284]

Sufentanil[126]	As an adjunct to other agents: 1–2 μg/kg IV. As the main anesthetic agent: 10–15 μg/kg IV. Half-life: 0.2–0.4 hr.[347]
Thiopental	7–8 mg/kg IV in infants. 4–6 mg/kg IV if the patient is older than 1 yr.[316] 15–20 mg/kg PR.

MUSCLE RELAXANTS

Atracurium	Intubating dose: 0.5 mg/kg IV. Onset: 2–4 mins. Duration: 20–45 mins. Time to 25% recovery after IV injection: approximately 30 mins.[249] Continuous use: bolus 0.1 mg/kg IV, then up to 5–10 μg/kg/min.[100] Monitor relaxation with a nerve stimulator. May cause histamine release with hypotension and flushing. Independent of renal or hepatic metabolism.
Cisatracurium[367]	0.15 mg/kg IV. Time to 100% block: 2 mins in infants; 3 mins in children. Time to 95% recovery of block: 65 mins in infants; 55 mins in children.
D-Tubocurarine	Intubating dose: 0.5 mg/kg IV.

Time to 50% recovery after IV injection: 45–65 mins.[249]

Doxacurium
Intubating dose: 30 μg/kg IV.[88]
Onset: 3–5 mins.
Time to 25% recovery after IV injection: approximately 30 mins.[249]
Duration: ≥60 mins.
Infusion: 10–14 μg/kg/min, but up to twice the dose may be needed.[247]
No cardiovascular effects.
Do not use doxacurium in neonates, because it contains benzyl alcohol, which may cause potentially fatal neurologic complications.

Mivacurium
Intubating dose: 0.2–0.3 mg/kg IV.[108]
Onset: 2–4 mins.
Time to 25% recovery after IV injection: approximately 6 mins.[249]
Recovery is fairly rapid (10–20 mins). Useful for short procedures and for intraoperative “wake-up” (e.g., during spinal fusion).
Infusion: 9–12 μg/kg/min (may vary from 3 to 24 μg/kg/min).[194]
Younger patients require higher infusion rates.[247]
Respiratory muscles are relaxed before the peripheral muscles.
Metabolized by pseudocholinesterase.

Pancuronium	Intubating dose: 0.1 mg/kg IV. Time to 10% recovery after IV injection: 25 mins.[249]
Pipecuronium[50]	Intubating dose: 40–50 μg/kg IV. Onset: 3–5 mins. Duration: ≥60 mins. Time to 10% recovery after IV injection: approximately 25 mins.[249] No cardiovascular effects.
Rapacuronium	Intubating dose: 2–3 mg/kg IV for children; 1–2 mg/kg IV for infants. Duration: 15–20 mins in children; 10–12 mins in infants.[16] Median effective dose: 0.78 mg/kg in children; 0.3 mg/kg in infants.[389,390]
Rocuronium[226]	Intubating dose: 0.6 mg/kg IV.[116] Onset: 90% neuromuscular block in 0.8 min; 100% neuromuscular block in 1.3 mins. Because of its rapid onset, rocuronium is most suited to rapid sequence induction (1.0–1.2 mg/kg IV). Median time to 25% recovery after IV injection: 41 mins (range, 24–68) in infants; 27 mins (range, 17–41) in children.[131] Duration: 20–45 mins. Maintenance infusion: 10–12 μg/kg/min.

	1.0 mg/kg IM in infants and 1.8 mg/kg into the deltoid muscle in children produce satisfactory intubating conditions in 2.5 mins in infants and in 3 mins in children; complete neuromuscular block is achieved in 5–6 mins in both groups.[292] No cardiovascular side effects.
Succinylcholine	Younger than 1 yr: 3 mg/kg IV[102]; 4 mg/kg IM (IM onset: 1.5–3.0 mins). 1 yr or older: 1 mg/kg IV; 2 mg/kg IM (IM onset: 1.5–3.0 mins). Time to 50% recovery after IV injection: 3.5–4.5 mins.[249] Duration after an IM injection: approximately 20 mins. Infusion: 7.5 mg/kg/hr. Tachyphylaxis starts after approximately 3 mg/kg total. Phase II block takes approximately 40 mins to wear off to a train-of-four of 75%. Monitor with a nerve stimulator. Contraindicated in patients who are undergoing reconstructive surgery after burns or massive trauma, those who have been confined to bed for more than a few days, and those who have a muscle disease;

	acute hyperkalemia (K^+ >5.5 mEq/L) may result.
Vecuronium	Intubating dose: 0.1 mg/kg IV. Onset: 2–4 mins. Reversible in approximately 15–30 mins after a usual intubating dose. Duration is 20–45 mins but in infants is significantly longer (much like that of pancuronium). Continuous use: bolus 250 μg/kg, then 1 μg/kg/min for infants (double this dose for children).[237] No cardiovascular effects. Depends on renal and hepatic elimination.

Notes

- Reduce doses of nondepolarizing relaxants by one-third in presence of halogenated agents, hypothermia, shock, acidosis, dehydration, prematurity, or certain antibiotics.
- Monitor the degree of neuromuscular blockade by peripheral nerve stimulator frequently; patient responses vary.
- Some of the above data are from D. M. Fisher.[362]

Infusion Requirements to Maintain 90–95% Neuromuscular Blockade

Drug	*Neonates*	*Infants*	*Children**	*Adults*
Atracurium (μg/kg/hr)	400	456	558	383
Mivacurium (μg/kg/hr)	—	—	780	360
Vecuronium (μg/kg/hr)	—	62	144	102

*All doses are under balanced anesthesia in children, except mivacurium, which is under halothane anesthesia.
Source: Modified from C. C. McLoughlin and R. K. Mirahkur.[237]

NOTES

NOTES

NOTES

3

Maintenance of Anesthesia

OPIOIDS*

Comparative Potencies

Equipotent doses in mg/kg[354]:

Morphine	1
Codeine	1.2
Fentanyl	0.01
Hydromorphone	0.015–0.020
Meperidine	0.1
Methadone	0.1
Oxycodone	0.15
Sufentanil	0.001

Dosages

Alfentanil — As the main anesthetic agent: 100 μg/kg IV followed by an average infusion rate of 2.4 μg/kg/min.[316]

*Narcotics are not advised for premature neonates younger than 60 wks (postconception) or for neonates (first month of life) unless they will be managed postoperatively in an intensive care unit.

	Half-life: 6–12 mins.[347] As a supplement to N_2O/O_2 general anesthesia: 20–25 μg/kg IV,[126] then an IV infusion of 1–3 μg/kg/min.[122] As adjunct to other agents: 20–25 μg/kg IV.[126]
Fentanyl	Induction: 10–15 μg/kg IV. Half-life: 2.0–3.5 hrs. Infusion: 2–4 μg/kg/hr[95]; titrate as needed. When inhalation agents are used, lower doses are adequate.
Meperidine	1.0–1.5 mg/kg IV single dose.[259] Half-life: 2–3 hrs.[347]
Morphine	10–30 μg/kg IV push. Infusion: for patients older than 5 yrs, load with up to 60 μg/kg IV. Titrate every 30 mins to a satisfactory rate, starting from 10–40 μg/kg/hr. Watch respiratory rate. Half-life: 3.9 hrs in children; 6.8 hrs in neonates.[100]
Sufentanil	1–2 μg/kg IV as a single dose to supplement N_2O.[126] Infusion: 1–3 μg/kg/min; neonates and infants younger than 3 mos: half this dose. Half-life: 0.2–0.4 hr.[347]

INTRAVENOUS AGENTS: INFUSIONS

Ketamine	Induction: 1–2 mg/kg IV. Maintenance infusion: 25–75 μg/kg/min.
Propofol	Infusion: 2 mg/kg IV for the initial bolus. Initial infusion: 60 μg/kg/hr; titrate as required.[100]
Thiopental	7–8 mg/kg IV in infants; 4–6 mg/kg IV if older than 1 yr.[316] Infusion: 5–10 mg/kg/hr.

NOTES

4

Reversal

DRUGS

Atropine	0.03 mg/kg IV before neostigmine. 0.015 mg/kg IV before edrophonium.
Doxapram	0.5–1.0 mg/kg IV. For neonatal apnea of prematurity: ≤3 mg/kg.[78] Maintenance: increments of 0.5–1.0 mg/kg/hr to a maximum of 2 mg/kg/hr if needed.
Edrophonium	1 mg/kg IV, preceded by atropine 0.015 mg/kg IV. Duration: approximately 1 hr.
Flumazenil	Increments of 0.01 mg/kg IV at 1-min intervals to a maximum of 0.2 mg/kg. Monitor for 1–2 hrs after because of the possibility of resedation.[91] Useful for intraoperative wake-up test during spinal fusion if patient has been sedated with midazolam.

	If no IV is in place, 0.4 mg/kg may be given PR.
	Effective in 10–15 mins.[236]
Glycopyrrolate	10 μg/kg IV.
Nalmefene	An alternative to naloxone.
	0.5–1.0 μg/kg IV q6–8h as needed.
Naloxone[4,118]	Neonates and children younger than 5 yrs and <20 kg: 10 μg/kg IV as a single dose; repeat in 2–5 mins as needed.
	Children older than 5 yrs: 0.4–2.0 mg IV; repeat in 2 mins if needed.
	Onset: <2 mins.
	Duration: approximately 45 mins.
	Infusion: 0.04–0.16 mg/kg/hr.
	Assess every 2 hrs as long as narcotic respiratory depression is a possibility, because the effect of the narcotic may outlast that of naloxone.
	May be given ET in an emergency.
Neostigmine	0.05–0.07 mg/kg IV preceded by atropine 0.03 mg/kg IV.
	Duration: approximately 1 hr.
Physostigmine	0.01–0.03 mg/kg/dose IV slowly.
	For reversal of tricyclic antidepressants and their side effects, such as seizures and dysrhythmias in children[203]; also for reversing the sialagogue and sedative effects of scopolamine.[382]

	Repeat in 15 mins for a maximum of four doses if needed. Infusion rate should be no higher than 0.5 mg/kg/min.
Protamine[271]	Give 1 mg protamine for every 100 units (1 mg) of remaining heparin activity as determined by the activated clotting time. Normal values for activated clotting time are 120–140 secs. Must be given slowly (over 10 mins or by infusion). Treat hypotension (less common and less severe in infants and children) with slow calcium gluconate, 10 mg/kg IV.
Pyridostigmine	0.25 mg/kg IV; for myasthenia gravis. Duration: approximately 1.5 hrs.
Vitamin K_1	1 mg total IM or IV for neonatal prophylaxis.

REVERSAL OF NEUROMUSCULAR BLOCKADE

If no response to a single twitch or the first of a train-of-four stimulus is observed, wait for it. *Do not attempt reversal.*

Indications of Adequate Reversal

- Babies mouth or chew on the tracheal tube, cough, and move actively.

- Sustained, spontaneous lifting of the baby's legs is an indication of good reversal.
- Older children can sustain head lift for 5 secs, open eyes widely, stick out tongue, and cough.
- Inspiratory force is near normal; vital capacity is near 90% of control.
- Maximum minute ventilation is near 90% of control.
- Nerve stimulator
    - Single twitch: 100% of control.
    - No tetanic fade (at 50 Hz for 5 secs).
    - No post-tetanic facilitation.

Resistance to Nondepolarizing Relaxants[97]

Eliminate the following as causes:

- Neurologic problems
    - Upper motor lesions
    - Multiple sclerosis
    - Disuse atrophy
- Thermal injury (e.g., burns)
- Anticonvulsant drugs
- Liver damage

Interaction of Antibiotics with Muscle Relaxants, Neostigmine, and Calcium

	Increase in neuromuscular block		*Antagonizer of block from antibiotic-nondepolarizer interaction*	
Antibiotic	*Nondepolarizers*	*Succinylcholine*	*Neostigmine*	*Calcium*
Neomycin	Yes	Yes	Usually	Usually
Streptomycin	Yes	Yes	Yes	Usually
Gentamicin	Yes	N/S	Sometimes	Yes
Kanamycin	Yes	Yes	Sometimes	Sometimes
Paromomycin	Yes	N/S	Yes	Yes
Viomycin	Yes	N/S	Yes	Yes
Polymyxin A	Yes	N/S	No	No
Polymyxin B	Yes	Yes	No*	No
Colistin	Yes	Yes	No	Sometimes
Tetracycline	Yes	No	Partially	Partially
Lincomycin	Yes	N/S	Partially	Partially
Clindamycin	Yes	N/S	Partially	Partially

N/S = not studied.
*Block augmented by neostigmine.
Source: Reprinted with permission from J. J. Savarese.[378]

Reversal of Warfarin Sodium (Coumadin) Therapy[388]

For elective surgery:

- Discontinue Coumadin 1–3 days preoperatively.
- Maintain anticoagulation with IV heparin, keeping activated clotting time to one-half of control value.
- Allow prothrombin time to return to within a few seconds of normal.
- Stop heparin 4–6 hrs before surgery.

- Start heparin 48 hrs postoperatively.
- Resume Coumadin 7–10 days postoperatively.

For emergency surgery:

- Replace coagulation factors with fresh-frozen plasma.
- Vitamin K if Coumadin reversal has no effect for 24 hrs.

NOTES

NOTES

5

Anesthesia-Related Drugs

ANALGESICS*

Acetaminophen	PO: 15–20 mg/kg q4h.[1] PR: First dose 30–40 mg/kg, then 20–25 mg/kg q4h.[1] Maximum dose per 24 hrs: 60 mg/kg. For long-term therapy, reduce doses by half.
Acetylsalicylic acid[178]	10–15 mg/kg q4–6h. Maximum dose per 24 hrs: 60 mg/kg. Caveat: Acetylsalicylic acid should be avoided, because the development of Reye's syndrome is associated with its use in febrile pediatric patients.[1]
Alphaprodine	0.4–0.6 mg/kg IV; 0.4–1.2 mg/kg SQ.

*Narcotics are not advised for premature neonates younger than 60 wks postconception or for neonates (first month of life) unless they will be managed postoperatively in an intensive care unit.

Codeine	0.5–1.0 mg/kg IM or PO. Repeat q4–6h. Maximum: 5 mg/dose. Do not use IV or if body weight <5 kg.
Demerol	See Meperidine.
Diclofenac	1 mg/kg PO[243]; 1–2 mg/kg IV q6–8h.[244]
Fentanyl[128]	As single dose or a loading dose: 1–2 μg/kg IV. Postoperative IV infusion: 0.5–4.0 μg/kg/hr. Postoperative epidural infusion: Initial dose of 2 μg/kg, then infuse at 0.5 μg/kg/hr. For painful procedures: 15–20 μg/kg as a lollipop 30 mins preoperatively.[223,302,308] Fentanyl transdermal patch is not recommended for children younger than 12 yrs.[131]
Hydromorphone[242]	15–20 μg/kg/dose IV slowly. Repeat to effect q3h. 75–100 μg/kg PO q3–4h. Half-life: 2–4 hrs.[347]
Ibuprofen	4–10 mg/kg PO q8h[308]; 40 mg/kg PR.[235] Maximum dose per 24 hrs: 40 mg/kg.

Indomethacin	For analgesia: 1.0 mg/kg q8h.[276] No more than three doses per day. Patent ductus closure: 0.2 mg/kg IV or PO q12h × three doses.[275]
Ketorolac[244]	0.5–1.0 mg/kg IV or IM q6h. Restrict use to short periods and minimal effective doses. Avoid using in patients with coagulopathy, nephropathy, or hypovolemia or in high-risk surgery. Ketorolac is equianalgesic with acetaminophen, but ketorolac is associated with more bleeding.[306] Provides good postoperative analgesia.[106]
Lorazepam	0.02–0.09 mg/kg IV.[308]
Meperidine	0.8–1.0 mg/kg IV q2h[244]; 1 mg/kg PO and IM q6h. Half-life: 2–3 hrs.[347] Infusion: 0.6 mg/kg/hr; titrate to requirements. Monitor vital signs closely. Not for long-term use.
Methadone	0.1 mg/kg IV, IM, or PO. Prolonged analgesia (12–36 hrs).[1] Half-life: 12–24 hrs.[347]
Midazolam sedation[313]	Postoperatively: Load with 80 μg/kg IV and increase to the

	desired effect. Maximum dose: 1 mg/kg.
	Infuse at 40–120 μg/kg/hr IV.
Morphine sulfate	Doses may require adjustment if the patient has been given morphine recently.
	The elimination half-life of morphine sulfate is 6.8 hrs in the first week of life and 3.9 hrs in older children[100]; in one study, however, it was found to be 13.9 hrs in neonates and 2 hrs in older children and adults.[105]
	IM: 0.1–0.2 mg/kg for premedication
	IV: 25 μg/kg if younger than 6 mos, and 50 μg/kg if older than 6 mos.
	Intrathecal: 20–30 μg/kg (preservative-free preparation).[42]
	Caudal epidural: 50–75 μg/kg (preservative-free preparation).[43]
	Lumbar epidural: 50 μg/kg (preservative-free preparation).[44]
	IV infusions
	Use a solution of 0.5 mg/kg morphine in 50 mL D5W.
	2 mL/hr of this solution will deliver 10 μg/kg/hr.[2,41]

	Postoperative ventilation[2,41] Loading dose: 100–150 µg/kg IV over 10 mins. Infuse at 10–15 µg/kg/hr IV; titrate as needed. Neonatal loading dose: 25–50 µg/kg IV. Infuse at 5–15 µg/kg/hr; titrate as needed. Spontaneous breathing[146] Loading dose: 150 µg/kg IV. Maintain the infusion at 5 µg/kg/hr if body weight is <10 kg, and at 10 µg/kg/hr if body weight is >10 kg. Close monitoring of vital signs is essential. Patient-controlled analgesia[96] See Patient-Controlled Analgesia. Subcutaneous infusion[184] Use a solution of MSO_4: 1 mg/kg in 20 mL saline. Place an SQ needle for pump infusion over deltoid muscle. Start the infusion after induction of anesthesia at 0.4 mL/hr. Postoperatively, continue at 0.5 mL/hr (up to 0.6 mL/hr for severe pain). Monitor closely.
Naprosyn	7 mg/kg PO q12h. No more than two doses/24 hrs.

Oxycodone	0.2 mg/kg PO.[1]
Paracetamol	10–20 mg/kg PO q6h. Do not use if patient is younger than 6 mos.
Pentazocine	0.2–0.3 mg/kg IV; 1 mg/kg IM.
Sufentanil	0.05 μg/kg IV. Nasally: 3 μg/kg.[245] Half-life: 0.2–0.4 hr.[347]

ANALGESICS AND SEDATIVES FOR NEONATES[285]

Chloral hydrate	Ideal for weaning from ventilator, because it does not alter chemoreceptor activity to CO_2 in newborns. Use <50 mg/kg PO.
Midazolam[313]	0.05–0.10 mg/kg IV followed by an infusion of 0.04 mg/kg/hr.
Morphine	0.1–0.2 mg/kg IV or IM followed q4h or, better still, by infusion at 10–20 μg/kg/hr titrated to response. Should be managed in an intensive care unit.
Fentanyl	Infusion of 1–5 μg/kg/hr is better than morphine for patients with labile pulmonary resistance. Add a 20-μg/kg bolus just before tracheal suction or physiotherapy.

PATIENT-CONTROLLED ANALGESIA

Children do best with a background infusion of IV morphine. In cases of patient-controlled analgesia for patients 5–17 yrs old, begin when the patient is "awake" enough to follow commands and express discomfort:

1. Establish a background IV infusion.
   MSO_4: 20 μg/kg/hr
   Fentanyl: 0.2 μg/kg/hr
   Hydromorphone: 4 μg/kg/hr
2. Set up patient-controlled analgesia system.
   Loading doses
      MSO_4: 50–100 μg/kg IV. Repeat prn × 5
      Fentanyl: 0.5–1.0 μg/kg q5min prn
      Hydromorphone: 10–20 μg/kg
   Each dose
      MSO_4: 20 μg/kg
      Fentanyl: 0.2 μg/kg
      Hydromorphone: 4 μg/kg
   Lockout interval
      MSO_4: 8–10 mins
      Fentanyl: 5–6 mins
      Hydromorphone: 8–10 mins
   4-hr limit setting
      MSO_4: approximately 300 μg/kg
      Fentanyl: 4–5 μg/kg
      Hydromorphone: 100 μg/kg

The respiratory depression effects of fentanyl last longer than its analgesic effects. Respiration rate and SaO_2 must be monitored after cessation of administration.

Figure 5.1.▶ Inadequate analgesia algorithm for morphine administered by patient-controlled anesthesia (PCA). Alternative analgesics are as follows: fentanyl 1 = morphine dose × 0.01 (e.g., 20 μg morphine = 0.2 μg fentanyl); hydromorphone = morphine dose × 0.2 (e.g., 20 μg morphine = 4 μg hydromorphone). (NSAIDs = nonsteroidal anti-inflammatory drugs.)

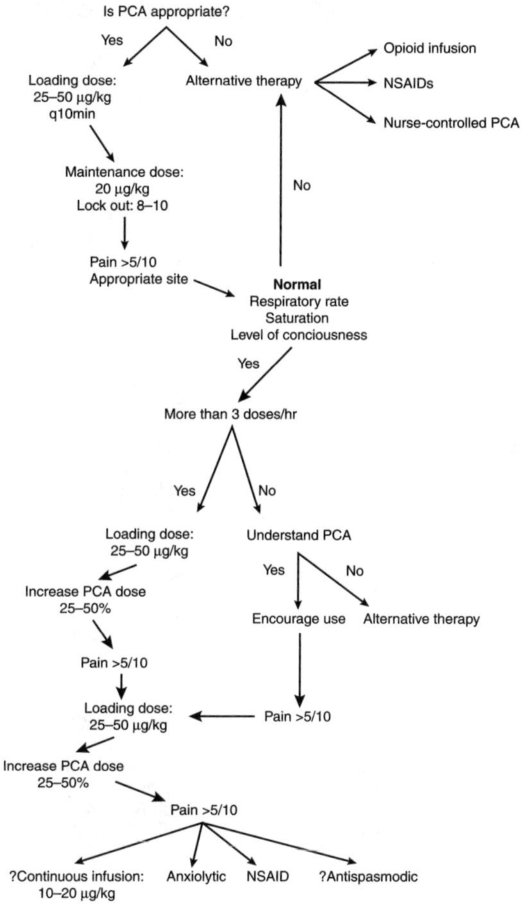
Is PCA appropriate?
Yes
No
Loading dose: 25–50 μg/kg q10min
Alternative therapy
Opioid infusion
NSAIDs
Nurse-controlled PCA
Maintenance dose: 20 μg/kg Lock out: 8–10
No
Pain >5/10 Appropriate site
Normal Respiratory rate Saturation Level of conciousness
Yes
More than 3 doses/hr
Yes
No
Loading dose: 25–50 μg/kg
Understand PCA
Yes
No
Increase PCA dose 25–50%
Encourage use
Alternative therapy
Pain >5/10
Loading dose: 25–50 μg/kg
Pain >5/10
Increase PCA dose 25–50%
Pain >5/10
?Continuous infusion: 10–20 μg/kg
Anxiolytic
NSAID
?Antispasmodic

ANTIBIOTICS FOR INFANTS AND CHILDREN[3]

Antibiotics that may need to be given preoperatively are listed below. See the next section for neonatal doses, which may differ.

Antibiotic	*Dose (mg/kg, except where noted)*	*Frequency and route*
Amikacin[110]	5.0–7.5	q8h IV or IM
Ampicillin[327]	50–100	q6h IV or IM
Carbenicillin[324]	75–100 (100–150)	q4h IV (q6h IM)
Cephalothin[324]	15–25	q4h IV
Cefaclor	12.5	q8h PO
Cefamandole[110]	12.5–40.0	q6h IV or IM
Cefazolin[110]	20–30	q8h IV or IM
Cefotaxime[110]	25–50	q12h IV or IM
Cefoxitin[110,324]	20–40	q6h IV
Ceftazidime[110]	30–50	q12h IV or IM
Cefuroxime[83]	25–50	q6h (for epiglottitis)
Ceftriaxone[110]	50	q12h IV
Cephalexin	6–12	q6h IV or IM
Cephalothin[332]	12.5–25.0	q4h IV or IM
Chloramphenicol[324]	25	q6h IV
Clindamycin[110]	8–12	q8h IV or IM
Cloxacillin[327]	12.5	q6h IV
Erythromycin[324]	3–5	q6h IV over 60 mins
Fluconazole[324]	3–6	q24h IV or PO
Gentamicin[324]	1.5–2.5	q8h IV over 20 mins or IM
Kanamycin[324]	3.0–7.5	q12h IV over 20 mins or IM
Methicillin[324]	50–100	q6h IV or IM
Metronidazole[327]	7.5	q6h IV
Nafcillin[327]	25–50	q6h IV or IM
Oxacillin[324]	25–50	q6h IV or IM
Penicillin G[324]	25,000–50,000 U	q4–6h IV or IM
Tetracycline HCl[332]	5–10	q12h
Tobramycin	2.5	q8h IV or IM
Vancomycin[332]	15–20	q8h IV over 45–60 mins

Source: References 3, 80, 110, 324, 327, and 332.

ANTIBIOTICS FOR NEONATES[3]

The following are antibiotics that may need to be given in the operating room. Doses are total daily doses in mg/kg/24 hrs and should be divided into the stated dose intervals.

		Weight of patient younger than 1 wk		*Weight of patient older than 1 wk*	
Drug	*Route*	*<2 kg*	*>2 kg*	*<2 kg*	*>2 kg*
Amikacin	IV, IM	7.5 q12h	10 q12h	10 q8h	10 q8h
Ampicillin[110]	IV, IM	50 q12h	50 q8h	50 q8h	50 q6h
Carbenicillin	IV, IM	100 q12h	100 q8h	100 q8h	100 q6h
Cefoxitin[110]	IV	40 q12h	40 q12h	40 q12h	40 q12h
Cefotaxime[110]	IV, IM	40 q12h	50 q12h	50 q8h	50 q8h
Ceftazidime[110]	IV, IM	100 q12h	100 q12h	100 q12h	100 q12h
Ceftriaxone[195]	IV, IM	50 q24h	50 q24h	50 q24h	75 q24h
Cefazolin[110]	IV, IM	40 q12h	40 q12h	40 q12h	40 q12h
Cephapirin[110]	IV	40 q12h	40 q12h	60 q12h	60 q12h
Cephalothin[195]	IV	20 q12h	20 q12h	20 q8h	20 q8h
Chloramphenicol[377]	IV[b]	2.5 q6h	5.0 q6h	25 q24h	25 q12h
Clindamycin[110,a]	IV, IM	15 q8h	15 q8h	15 q8h	15 q8h
Erythromycin[377]	IV, IM	10 q12h	15 q12h	15 q12h	20 q12h
Gentamicin	IV, IM	2.5 q18h[195]	2.5 q12h	2.5 q8h	2.5 q8h
Kanamycin	IV, IM	7.5 q12h	10 q12h	7.5 q8h	10 q8h
Methicillin	IV, IM	25 q12h	25 q8h	25 q8h	25 q6h
Metronidazole	IV	7.5 q48h	7.5 q24h	7.5 q12h	7.5 q12h[195]
Moxalactam	IV, IM	50 q12h	50 q8h	50 q8h	50 q8h
Nafcillin	IV, IM	25 q12h	25 q8h	25 q8h	25 q6h
Oxacillin	IV	25 q12h	25 q8h	25 q8h	25 q6h
Penicillin G	IM	75,000 U	q12h	75,000 U	q6–8h
Tobramycin	IV, IM	2 q12h	2 q12h	2 q8h	2 q8h
Vancomycin[a,b]	IV	10 q12h	10 q12h	10 q8h	10 q8h

[a]Serum drug concentrations should be monitored for these antibiotics.

[b]Vancomycin should always be administered as a slow IV infusion over 60 mins. Allergic reactions can be severe, especially when the dose is administered too quickly. Diphenhydramine (Benadryl), 1 mg/kg, is the best antihistaminic; steroids and circulatory support may be needed.

ANTICONVULSANTS

Diazepam	0.1–0.3 mg/kg IV at 1 mg/min to a maximum of 10 mg. If no effect occurs in 15 mins, increase the dose to 0.25–0.40 mg/kg. Maximum total dose: 5 mg if younger than 5 yrs; 10 mg if older than 5 yrs.
Paraldehyde	IM: 0.15 mL/kg as a sedative, 0.30 mL/kg q2–4h for seizures. PR: 0.3–0.4 mL/mg as a 1:10 solution in oil. Maximum PR dose is 7 mL of this solution.
Phenobarbital[258]	For seizures: 15–20 mg/kg in a single dose or in divided doses. Maximum dose: 20 mg/kg. Maintenance dose: 2–4 mg/kg IV, IM, or PO q12h.
Phenytoin[324]	Loading dose: 1–3 mg/kg/min IV over 20 mins. Monitoring the ECG is essential while doing this. Maintenance dose: 2.5 mg/kg q12h IV or PO. Do not mix with other IV solutions. Note: Doses for cardiac dysrhythmias differ from these (see Cardioactive Drugs).
Thiopental	7–8 mg/kg IV in infants; 4–6 mg/kg if older than 1 yr.[316] Infuse at 5–10 mg/kg/hr.

ANTIHYPERTENSIVES

See the section on Vasodilators and Antihypertensives.

BRONCHODILATORS AND DECONGESTANTS

Albuterol[131]	Two aerosol inhalations if older than 4 yrs. Repeat q4–6h.
Aminophylline[268]	Loading dose up to 6 mg/kg slowly over 20–30 mins. Monitor heart rate and rhythm while doing this. IV infusion: for neonate, 0.2 mg/kg/hr; for younger than 1 yr, 0.2 mg/kg/hr; for ages 1–9 yrs, 1.0 mg/kg/hr. Half-life: in neonates, 30 hrs[124]; in children, 3–10 hrs.[139] PO: 5 mg/kg, then 3 mg/kg q8h. Therapeutic serum level: 10–20 μg/mL and a bolus dose of 1 mg/kg usually raise the serum level by 2 μg/mL.[349]
Atropine[314]	0.01 mg/kg IV; 0.02 mg/kg IM and PO. As an aerosol: 0.05 mg/kg/dose with a minimum of 0.25 mg and a maximum of 1 mg in 2–3 mL of normal saline, q6–8h.
Cocaine (4%)	1.0 mg/kg topically to the mucosa of the mouth, nose, or larynx only.[261]

Epinephrine[262]	10 μg/kg/min IV very slowly. Monitor heart rate and rhythm while doing this. May repeat in 20 mins if indicated. Infusion: 0.1–1.0 μg/kg/min.
Isoetharine[263]	Use 0.1 mL/kg of a 1% solution in 3 mL saline. Nebulize q2–6h. Maximum dose: 0.5 mL/kg.
Isoproterenol[250,273]	0.1 μg/kg/min by infusion, increasing slowly if needed. Stop if tachycardia exceeds 200/min. Because isoproterenol may cause significant tachycardia, aminophylline or terbutaline is preferred for bronchodilation. Isoproterenol may be used for severe asthma, which should be monitored (ECG and blood pressure) in an intensive care unit.[348] Can be given intratracheally or by aerosol inhalation.
Metaproterenol[264]	Use 0.1–0.2 mL/kg of a 5% solution. Minimum dose: 0.1 mL. Maximum dose: 0.3 mL of the 5% solution in 2–3 mL saline by nebulizer.
Methylprednisolone	For severe bronchospasm: 2–4 mg/kg/dose IV q4–6h.[324]

Racemic epinephrine	Add 0.5 mL of a 2.25% solution to 2–3 mL saline.[314] Aerosolize by micronebulizer q1–2h. Dose of the solution: patients who weigh <10 kg, 0.25 mL[307]; patients who weigh 20–40 kg, 0.5 mL; patients who weigh >40 kg, 0.75 mL.
Terbutaline	Jet nebulizer: Use a 0.1% solution and give 3 mL over 3 mins. Subcutaneous injection: 5–10 µg/kg. IV: 0.4 µg/kg/min increasing to a dose of 3–6 µg/kg/min.[314] Stop if tachycardia becomes a concern.

CARDIOACTIVE DRUGS

Adenosine[74,324,360]	100-µg/kg IV rapid bolus followed *immediately* by a bolus of 2–3 mL of normal saline to avoid sequestration of the drug into red blood cells before it reaches the heart. Increase the dose to 200 µg/kg/dose if the first dose is ineffective in 1–2 mins. Maximum total: 250 µg/kg.[258] For supraventricular tachycardia. A case report cites 200 µg/kg as an initial dose, repeated at 1–2 mins to the desired outcome.[66] May cause bronchospasm.

	Synchronized cardioversion (0.25–1.00 J/kg) if severe hemodynamic compromise occurs.[218]
Amiodarone[358,359]	Bolus: 1 mg/kg given over 5 mins and repeated five times to a maximum of 5 mg/kg. Infusion: 10–15 mg/kg/day (0.4–0.6 mg/kg/hr). Monitor for hypertension. For life-threatening ventricular tachyarrhythmias.
Amrinone	Load with 0.75 mg/kg over 2–3 mins.[265] Repeat in 30 mins prn. Follow with an infusion of 5–10 μg/kg/min, or 3–5 μg/kg/min in neonates.[47] Half-life: approximately 4.6 hrs.
Atropine	0.01 mg/kg IV; 0.02 mg/kg IM or PO. May be given intratracheally using 2.0–2.5 times the IV dose.
Bretylium	5 mg/kg IV slowly.[103] Repeat q10min if needed, to a maximum dose of 30 mg/kg.[5,76] Infusion: 15–30 μg/kg/min. For ventricular fibrillation or unstable ventricular tachycardia.
Calcium chloride (10%)[4]	For management of hypocalcemia, hypokalemia, and calcium-channel blocker overdose.

	Not recommended for treatment of asystole or electromechanical dissociation. Dose: 0.20–0.25 mL/kg infused slowly and repeated once after 10 mins if necessary. Check serum ionized calcium.
Defibrillation	See Chapter 15.
Dextrose and insulin	For inotropy: add 12.5 U soluble insulin to 50 mL of 50% dextrose in water. Give a bolus of 0.5 mL/kg. For acute hyperkalemia (K^+ >5.5 mEq/L): add 5 U plain insulin to 20 mL 50% dextrose in water. Give 1 mL/kg IV and titrate if necessary.[171]
Diazoxide	Maximum initial dose: 5 mg/kg IV as slow bolus. Repeat in 45–60 mins if needed.
Digoxin (Lanoxin)	Total IV digitizing dose (with normal renal function) Premature: 15 μg/kg (lean body weight) IV. Full-term: 20 μg/kg (lean body weight) IV. Age 1–24 mos: 30 μg/kg (lean body weight) IV. Age 2–5 yrs: 20–30 μg/kg (lean body weight) IV. Age 5–10 yrs: 15–30 μg/kg (lean body weight) IV.

	Initial dose is one-third of total dose, the second dose (also one-third of total dose) is given 12 hrs later, and the third dose (the remaining one-third of total dose) is given 24 hrs after first dose. Oral doses are one-third more than IV doses. Monitor the serum levels, and check the ECG 6 hrs after each dose. Therapeutic serum level: 1.0–3.5 ng/mL. Excretion may be slow.
Diltiazem[131]	0.25-mg/kg IV bolus over 2 mins. Wait 15 mins; if the response is inadequate, give 0.35 mg/kg over 2 mins. Infusion: 2.0–3.5 μg/kg/min, although 1 μg/kg may be enough. Based on the adult dose; no pediatric IV dose is available.
Dobutamine[376]	An inotrope that has selective beta-adrenergic effects. Effect on blood pressure is variable. Titrate 2–20 μg/kg/min.
Dopamine[376]	1–3 μg/kg/min results in renal and splanchnic effects, mainly vasodilation of the renal vasculature. 5–10 μg/kg/min results in inotropic effects.

	10–20 μg/kg/min causes inotropic, chronotropic, and vasoconstrictive effects. Adjust rate as needed. More than 20 μg/kg/min results in no additional benefit.
Ephedrine	0.2–0.3 mg/kg IV. Maximum dose is 0.5 mg.[259]
Epinephrine[4,251,259,266]	Note: Two different concentrations of epinephrine solutions are needed for recommended doses. The 1:1,000 solution contains 1 mg/mL; the 1:10,000 solution contains 0.1 mg/mL. Take care to use the appropriate concentrations. Hypotension: 2–4 μg/kg IV as a push repeated as needed or followed by an IV infusion at 0.1–1.0 μg/kg/min, titrating as needed. For symptomatic bradycardia: 0.01 mg/kg (0.1 mL of the 1:10,000 solution) IV or IO. For ET administration: 0.1 mL/kg of the 1:1,000 solution IV or IO. Dilute with 3–5 mL saline, and follow with approximately 5 mL saline flush and then a few deep positive pressure breaths. For neonates, use the 1:10,000 solution for ET administration.

	For pulseless arrest: 0.01 mg/kg (0.1 mL of the 1:10,000 solution) IV or IO. If no response, subsequent doses are increased to 0.1 mg/kg (0.1 mL/kg of the 1:1,000 solution). Repeat every 3–5 mins during arrest. Doses as high as 0.2 mg/kg may be beneficial.[8] If the condition persists, a high-dose infusion of 20 μg/kg/min may be commenced and reduced when an effective pulse has returned.[179]
	For infusion: Start with 0.1–0.2 μg/kg/min. Titrate as needed. Maximum: 1.0 μg/kg/min. Usually, <0.3 μg/kg/min results in alpha effects, and >0.3 μg/kg/min results in beta effects.
Esmolol[92]	0.5–1.0 mg/kg/min slowly over 1–2 mins (beta blocker).
	Follow the above dose with 50–200 μg/kg/min. Titrate to desired effect. Useful for controlled hypotension.
Glycopyrrolate[267]	5–10 μg/kg IV; 10 μg/kg IM.
Isoproterenol[4,273]	0.1 μg/kg/min by infusion to start.
	Useful for nodal bradycardia, atrioventricular dissociation with slow response, and bradycardia not responding to atropine.
	Can be given intratracheally using 2.0–2.5 times the usual dose.

Drug	Dose and notes
Labetalol[149]	0.25 mg/kg IV initially. Onset is rapid. Repeat double this dose q15min if necessary. Maximum total cumulative dose of 1.75 mg/kg. Can be given as an infusion of 1–3 mg/kg/hr. An alpha and beta blocker. Half-life: 5–8 hrs.
Lidocaine[259]	1-mg/kg bolus IV q5min. Maximum total dose: 5 mg/kg. Then 20–50 µg/kg/min by infusion. Can be given intratracheally using 2.0–2.5 times the usual dose.
Norepinephrine	0.05–1.00 µg/kg/min by infusion.[211] Maximum dose: 1–2 µg/kg/min.
Phenylephrine[259]	5–20 µg/kg IV; 0.1 mg/kg IM. Infusion: 0.1–0.5 µg/kg/min IV. For hypotension from low systemic vascular resistance.
Phenytoin[144]	Loading dose: 2.5 mg/kg IV over 10 mins. Repeat q15min if necessary, to a total of 10 mg/kg. For ventricular tachycardia or dysrhythmias due to digitalis[150] or due to bupivacaine[136,198] toxicity. Monitor the ECG.
Procainamide	Loading dose: 7–15 mg/kg IV very slowly over 30 mins.[4,259] Use half this dose for infants.

	Infusion: 20–60 μg/kg/min. Monitor blood pressure and heart rate. For refractory symptomatic ventricular tachycardia.
Propranolol	10–25 μg/kg/dose slowly IV q10min.[4,76] May repeat q5–10min if necessary. Maximum: Four doses. For atrial tachydysrhythmia. Contraindicated in asthmatics.
Quinidine	15–30 mg quinidine base/kg/day PO divided q4–6h.[260]
Verapamil[5]	For younger than 1 yr: 0.1–0.2 mg/kg IV over 2 mins. For ages 1–15 yrs: 0.1–0.3 mg/kg over 2 mins. Give over 2 mins. Maximum: three doses at intervals of 15–30 mins. Monitor ECG. Useful for supraventricular tachydysrhythmia. Be especially careful with infants younger than 1 yr in whom hypotension and circulatory collapse have been reported. Contraindicated in Wolff-Parkinson-White syndrome.

COAGULANTS: AGONISTS AND ANTAGONISTS

Aminocaproic acid	100 mg/kg IV slow push, then 33 mg/kg/hr.[269]
Heparin[270]	50- to 100-U/kg IV initial bolus (1 mg = 100 U). Follow with continuous infusion, 10–25 U/kg/hr, or intermittent IV, 100 units/kg q4h. Monitor the effect using the ACT test. Normal = 90–120 secs.
Protamine sulfate	Give 1.0–1.3 mg protamine for every 100 U (1 mg) of heparin given in previous 2 hrs.[271] Repeat as indicated by laboratory data (ACT). Protamine causes vasodilation and hypotension; it must be given slowly (infusion). Treat hypotension with calcium gluconate, 10 mg/kg IV.
Vitamin K_1[272]	Infants: 1–2 mg/kg IM or IV. Children: 5–10 mg/kg IV. Onset: 2–3 hrs.

DIURETICS

Chlorothiazide	10–15 mg/kg q12h PO.
Ethacrynic acid	1 mg/kg IV. Onset in 5 mins; peaks in 45 mins.
Furosemide	1 mg/kg IV. Onset in 5 mins; peaks in 30 mins.
Hydrochlorothiazide	1.5 mg/kg q12h PO.
Mannitol	0.5–1.0 g/kg IV over 20–30 mins. For neurosurgery: 2 g/kg IV over 20–30 mins.
Spironolactone	1–2 mg/kg/day PO divided into q4–8h. Peaks in days.

MISCELLANEOUS DRUGS

Caffeine	5–10 mg/kg IV for apnea in full-term and premature neonates.[75,77,125]
Dextrose (10%)	For asymptomatic hypoglycemia: 4.0 mg/kg/kg IV.[259] For symptomatic hypoglycemia: See Chapter 12.
Glucagon[278]	Younger than 5 yrs: 0.5 mg/dose SQ or IM. Older than 5 yrs: 1.0 mg/dose SQ or IM. Monitor serum glucose.

	Maximum dose: 1 mg. Keep dextrose infusion running while awaiting effect of glucagon.
Magnesium SO_4[163]	25 mg/kg q4–6h for three to four doses maximum. Use 50% solution for IM and a 1% solution for IV. Calcium gluconate is the antidote.
Methylene blue[277]	For methemoglobinemia: 1–2 mg/kg IV. Repeat in 1 hr if needed.
Prostaglandin E_1[279]	To maintain the patency of ductus: 0.1 μg/kg IV or intra-arterial. Infusion: 0.1 μg/kg/min IV. Maximum, 0.4 mg/kg/min. Monitor for apnea, hypotension, and hypoglycemia, and maintain adequate intravascular volume.

STEROIDS

Dexamethasone	0.5 mg/kg IV (maximum total: 4.0).
Hydrocortisone	1 mg/kg IV q6h.[203]
Methylprednisolone	2–4 mg/kg IV q4–6h. For massive CNS trauma: 30 mg/kg IV, then 5.6 mg/kg/hr.

Relative Potency[200]

Steroid	*Anti-inflammatory properties**	*Mineralo-corticoid*	*Equivalent dose (mg)*	*Half-life (hrs)*
Hydrocortisone	1	1	20	8
Cortisone	0.8	0.8	25	—
Prednisone	4	0.25	5	12–36
Prednisolone	4	0.25	5	—
Methylprednisolone	5	—	4	20
Triamcinolone	5	—	4	—
Dexamethasone	30	—	0.75	36–54

*Relative milligram comparisons with cortisol. Glucocorticoid and mineralocorticoid properties are set as 1.

Source: Reprinted with permission from G. Graf and S. Rosenbaum.[200]

SYMPATHOMIMETICS

The adrenergic effects of catecholamines are as follows:

Catecholamine	*Beta$_1$*	*Beta$_2$*	*Alpha*	*Dopamine*
Dopamine	++	+	+	+++
Dobutamine	+++	+	+	—
Isoproterenol	++++	++++	0	—
Epinephrine	++	0	+++	—
Norepinephrine	++	0	++++	—

Source: Reprinted with permission from D. Hatch et al.[217]

Drugs

Dobutamine

Start with 3 µg/kg/min by infusion.
Range: 2–10 µg/kg/min causes beta$_1$ and beta$_2$ effects; >10 µg/kg/min causes alpha and beta effects.
Half-life: approximately 2 mins.

Dopamine	1–3 μg/kg/min results in renal and splanchnic effects, mainly vasodilation in the renal vasculature. 5–10 μg/kg/min results in inotropic effects. Adjust rates as needed. 10–20 μg/kg/min results in inotropic, chronotropic, and vasoconstrictive effects. More than 20 μg/kg/min results in no additional benefit.
Ephedrine	0.2–0.3 mg/kg IV. Maximum dose: 0.5 mg.[259]
Epinephrine[251,259,266]	1:10,000 solution contains 100 μg/mL. For hypotension: 2–4 μg/kg; 0.1–1.0 μg/kg/min IV, titrating as needed. For profound bradycardia or anaphylaxis: 10 μg/kg IV or IO q3–5min as needed. ET: 2.0–2.5 times this dose; inject beyond the distal end of the ET tube (catheter) and follow with a 5-mL saline flush and several positive-pressure breaths. Half-life: 1.5–2.0 mins.

	For surgical infiltration: With enflurane or isoflurane, ≤30 μg/kg/dose.
	With halothane and normocapnia: ≤5 μg/kg/dose. Minimum intervals between doses: 20 mins.
	For edema of airway: Racemic epinephrine (2.25%), 2–4 mL, in saline. Nebulize q30min.
	For cardiac arrest: See Chapter 15.
Isoproterenol[273]	0.1 μg/kg/min by infusion to start with. Titrate to effect.
Norepinephrine	0.05–1.00 μg/kg/min by infusion.[149,211]
Phenylephrine[259]	IV: 5–20 μg/kg; IM: 0.1 mg/kg. Infusion: 0.1–0.5 μg/kg/min IV. For hypotension from low systemic vascular resistance.

VASODILATORS AND ANTIHYPERTENSIVES

Captopril	10–40 μg/kg PO q6–8h. Maximum daily total: 5 mg. For facilitating controlled hypotension: 0.3 mg/kg PO, 1.5 hr preoperatively.
Chlorpromazine	0.25 mg/kg/dose IV slowly.
Diazoxide	1–3 mg/kg (lean body weight) IV push.

	Give half this dose if patient is also taking other antihypertensives. Maximum dose: 5 mg. Repeat in 45–60 mins if needed. Effect lasts 3–15 hrs.
Esmolol	0.5 mg/kg IV slowly over 1–2 mins[92] (beta blocker). Follow with 50–200 μg/kg/min by infusion and titrate to desired effect.[255]
Labetalol[149]	0.25 mg/kg IV initially. Onset is rapid. Repeat double this dose q15min if necessary. Maximum total cumulative dose of 1.75 mg/kg. Can be given as an infusion of 1–3 mg/kg/hr. Labetalol is an alpha and beta blocker with a half-life of 5–8 hrs.
Nifedipine[149]	0.25–0.50 mg/kg sublingually or PO. Onset is in 15–30 mins. Nifedipine is a calcium-channel blocker. Experience in children is limited.
Nitroglycerin	1–10 μg/kg/min by infusion. Half this dose for neonates.

Nitroprusside[259]	Administer by a separate infusion line. Start at <0.5 μg/kg/min by infusion. Maximum rate: for neonates, 6 μg/kg/min; for others, 10 μg/kg/min. Maximum total: 1.5 mg/kg over 4 hrs. Captopril, beta blockers, and inhalational anesthetic agents reduce nitroprusside requirements and control tachycardia. Be aware of thiocyanate toxicity (overdose, prolonged administration, and renal insufficiency). Signs of thiosulfate toxicity[292,293]: • Increasing requirements for sodium nitroprusside • Progressive hypotension that does not respond to fluids and vasopressors but that responds to sodium thiosulfate • Narrow pulse pressure • Metabolic acidosis • Bright red blood To prepare nitroprusside solution: Multiply weight (kg) by 10. Put this number of μg into each 1 mL of infusion fluid.

	This provides 10 μg/kg/min when infused at 1 mL/min.
	Antidotes[214]:
	Administer oxygen 100%.
	Sodium thiosulfate, 150 mg/kg IV.
	Sodium nitrite, 10 mg/kg IV initially, then 5 mg/kg over 30 mins.
	Hydroxocobalamin: IV 0.1 mg/kg.
	Correct acidosis, guided by arterial blood gases.
	Consider inhalation of amyl nitrate for 30 secs every 2 mins.
	Calcium chloride (10%) infusion may counter refractory hypotension. The dose is 0.20–0.25 mL/kg infused *slowly* and repeated once after 10 mins if necessary.[4] Check serum ionized calcium.
Phentolamine	30 μg/kg IV and repeat to desired effect.
	Maximum IV dose: 125 μg/kg.
	Infusion: 20 μg/kg/min.
	Usually used for management of pheochromocytoma.
Propranolol	10–25 μg/kg/dose slowly IV q10min.[4,76]

	Maximum: Four doses. Monitor ECG (bradycardia) and blood pressure. Propranolol is a beta blocker. Do not use for patients with asthma.
Tolazoline	0.25 mg/kg IV slowly via an arm or a scalp vein. Monitor for systemic hypotension. Tolazoline is an alpha blocker with a doubtful effect on pulmonary hypertension. Pulmonary artery bolus: 1 mg/kg slowly. Infusion: after loading with 1 mg/kg, infuse at 1–2 mg/kg/hr.
Trimethaphan	Infusion solution of 1.0 mg/mL. Start at 0.5 mg/min and titrate to effect.

VASOACTIVE INFUSIONS

Vasoactive infusions are used for children with body weight less than 25 kg. Administer by microdrip (60 drops = 1 mL).

Recommended doses[4,5] for these drugs are as follows:

Dopamine	1–3 μg/kg/min results in renal and splanchnic effects, mainly vasodilation in the renal vasculature.

Drug	Dosage
	5–10 μg/kg/min results in inotropic effects. Adjust rates as needed. 10–20 μg/kg/min results in inotropic, chronotropic, and vasoconstrictive effects. More than 20 μg/kg/min results in no additional benefit.
Dobutamine	Start with 3 μg/kg/min by infusion. Range: 2–10 μg/kg/min results in $beta_1$ and $beta_2$ effects. Above 10 μg/kg/min results in both alpha and beta effects.
Epinephrine	0.1–1.0 μg/kg/min. See Chapter 15 for specific applications.
Isoproterenol	0.1–1.0 μg/kg/min.
Lidocaine	20–50 μg/kg/min.[259]
Norepinephrine	0.1–0.5 μg/kg/min.
Nitroprusside	0.5–10.0 μg/kg/min. Maximum for neonates: 6 μg/kg/min.[259] Be aware of thiocyanate toxicity (overdose, prolonged administration, and renal insufficiency).

How to Make Infusion Solutions[98]

Administer by microdrip only (60 drops = 1 mL).

Drug and its concentration as supplied	*mL to be added to the carrier solution*	*Carrier solution*	*µg/kg/min delivered by an infusion rate of 1 mL/hr*
Dobutamine (12.5 mg/mL)	Weight × 1.2 mL	250 mL D5 ¼ NS	1
Dopamine (40 mg/mL)	Weight × 0.375 mL	250 mL D5 ¼ NS	1
Epinephrine (1 mg/mL)	Weight × 0.09 mL	250 mL D5 ¼ NS	0.006
Isoproterenol (0.2 mg/mL)	Weight × 0.45 mL	250 mL D5 ¼ NS	0.006
Nitroprusside (25 mg/mL)	Weight × 0.15 mL	250 mL D5W	0.25
Norepinephrine (1 mg/mL)	Weight × 0.09 mL	250 mL D5 ¼ NS	0.006
Phenylephrine (10 mg/mL)	Weight × 0.05 mL	250 mL D5 ¼ NS	0.033
Lidocaine (40 mg/mL)	Weight × 1.5 mL	250 mL D5 ¼ NS	4

NS = normal saline.

NOTES

NOTES

NOTES

NOTES

6

Monitoring the Pediatric Patient

BASIC REQUIREMENTS

Vital Patient observation is the most important monitoring modality. Use your senses (e.g., sight, touch, hearing, and *common sense*).

Essential Precordial stethoscope.

ECG.

Arterial blood pressure measurement: sphygmomanometer, Dinamap, doppler, arterial line.

Body temperature measurement.

A pulse oximeter for Hb saturation is essential.

Capnography for end-tidal CO_2 is required by American Society of Anesthesiologists guidelines[173] and by some states.

Peripheral nerve stimulator when muscle relaxants are used.

Optional Invasive arterial blood pressure (right radial artery is preductal).

Central venous pressure line.

Catheter for urine output.

Blood loss.

Equipment In-line sensor in the circuit's inspiratory breathing line for monitoring inspired O_2 concentration is mandatory.
High-low pressure alarm in the ventilator's breathing circuit is mandatory.
Check warming equipment frequently.

BLOOD PRESSURE MEASUREMENT

Use the width (not the length) of the blood pressure cuff to determine the correct size.

The width: ↑↓

The optimal cuff width–to–limb circumference ratio is 0.4 to 0.6.[72] Thus, the width of the cuff should be approximately equal to half the circumference of the limb (arm or leg) at the application site. Achieving this ratio exactly is not always possible; settle for a "best fit." Too large a cuff results in an artificially low reading; too small a cuff results in an artificially high reading. Oscillometric finger cuffs are suitable for monitoring systolic blood pressure in children and young adults.[216]

When using a cuff, the mean arterial pressure is calculated as follows:

$$\frac{(\text{Diastolic pressure} \times 2) + \text{systolic pressure}}{3}$$

Blood Pressures in the Normal Neonate

	Birth weight			
	<1 kg	*1–2 kg*	*2–3 kg*	*>3 kg*
Systolic pressure (mm Hg)	40–60	50–65	50–70	50–80
Diastolic pressure (mm Hg)	15–35	20–40	25–45	30–50

Note: Midarm and midcalf blood pressures in the neonate are identical.

MONITORING NEUROMUSCULAR BLOCKADE

After giving a nondepolarizing relaxant at induction of anesthesia:

- When the single twitch falls to 5% of control:
  —Intubating conditions are good.
  —Abdominal relaxation is good.
- When the neuromuscular block is intense:
  —There is no response to any electrical stimulus, and you do not know when the neuromuscular block will become "reversible"—that is, the point at which a response to a single non-facilitated stimulus will be seen.

The PTC provides this information:

1. The nerve stimulator must have been off for 30 seconds.
2. Apply a supramaximal tetanic stimulus: 50 Hz for 5 seconds.
3. Three seconds later, apply 1 Hz (once per second) stimuli, and count the number of responses seen or felt. These are "facilitated" or posttetanic responses.

4. The table indicates how long it will be before the block becomes "reversible." Note that the time intervals vary with the relaxant being used.
5. If you wish to repeat the test, wait for at least a minute with the stimulator turned off before doing so.

Time to the First Response to a Train-of-Four Stimulus

Post-tetanic count	Pancuronium[12,13]	Vecuronium[14]	Atracurium[15]
1	36 mins	8.5 mins	9 mins
2	25 mins	7 mins	7 mins
3	6 mins	—	5 mins
4	18 mins	5 mins	4 mins
5	—	4 mins	3 mins
6	10 mins	3 mins	2 mins
7	—	—	1 min
8	5 mins	2 mins	Imminent
9	—	—	1 min
10	Imminent	Imminent	—

Toward the End of Anesthesia

When the single twitch returns to 25% of control:

- The abdominal muscles will be tight.
- Only the first three of the TOF responses will be seen, and thus the TOF ratio will be zero.

NOTES

NOTES

7

Pediatric Airway

An in-depth discussion of the pediatric airway is provided in Riazi.[309]

NORMAL PEDIATRIC AIRWAY

- The buccal cavity is small, because the rami of the mandible are undeveloped.
- The tongue is relatively large because of the small buccal cavity.
- The larynx is high (at the C2 or C3 level) and tends to be tucked away under the base of the tongue.
- The epiglottis is omega-shaped (Ω) and soft and has a small base; these features make it "floppy."
- The smallest diameter is at the cricoid ring (in adults, it is at the vocal cords).
- The occiput is prominent; a small pillow or padding under the shoulders may be required for optimal positioning of the head.
- At approximately age 8 yrs, airway features are similar to those of an adult but smaller.

LARYNGEAL MASK AIRWAY[54]

Guide to Appropriate Use

Weight (kg)	*Laryngeal mask airway size*	*Cuff volume (mL)*
<6.5	1	2–5
6.5–20.0	2	7–10
20–30	2.5	14
30–70	3	15–20
>70	4	25–30

Note: Since this table was published, more sizes have been added: 3.5, 4.5, and 5. An intubating laryngeal mask airway is also available in three sizes: 3, 4, and 5. None of these is suitable for small patients; the smallest (size 3) is suitable for an adolescent.
Source: Modified with permission from S. Lowe and S. Hershey.[381]

A more sensible way to inflate the cuff is to inject enough air to seat the mask snugly in the pharynx or, if desired, to seal the leak when positive pressure is applied to the airway.

Awake insertion can be achieved as follows: Spray the hypopharynx and larynx with 2% lidocaine, and apply 2% viscous lidocaine to the mask. Insert the mask gently and induce anesthesia. The trachea can then be intubated by passing a fiberoptic laryngoscope of appropriate size with a tracheal tube over it through the laryngeal mask. When the larynx is seen, slide the tube into the trachea. This technique is especially useful for patients with difficult airways (as, for example, those with Pierre-Robin syndrome).[17]

The laryngeal mask airway does not prevent aspiration; this should be kept in mind in patients with risk factors for regurgitation.

Pennant and White[332] provide a detailed description of the laryngeal mask airway and its uses.

TRACHEAL TUBES

Cuffed or Uncuffed?

For patients up to age 8 yrs, use an uncuffed tube; for patients older than 8 yrs, use a cuffed tube.

Size

An audible leak should be present when a pressure of 20 cm H_2O is applied to the breathing circuit after intubation with an uncuffed tube. Expired CO_2 must be identified.[173]

When choosing a reinforced (armor) tube, select a tube one size smaller than the size suggested, because the walls of these tubes are thicker and thus increase the external diameter; this also applies when intubation for epiglottitis is planned.

<2 kg	2.5 mm internal diameter; uncuffed.
2.0–3.5 kg	3 mm internal diameter; uncuffed.
>3.5 kg	3.5 mm internal diameter; uncuffed.
6 mos old	4 mm internal diameter; uncuffed.
1 yr old	4.5 mm internal diameter; uncuffed.
Older than 2 yrs	Use the following formula: $\frac{\text{Age}}{4} + 4.5$ mm internal diameter
Older than 8 yrs	Use a cuffed tube with a leak as described.

Recommendations for Size and Type of Tracheal Tube

Age	*Size (mm ID)*	*Type*
Premature neonate	2.5–3.0	Uncuffed
Full-term neonate	3.0–3.5	Uncuffed
3 mos to 1 yr	4	Cuffed or uncuffed
2 yrs	4.5	Cuffed or uncuffed
4 yrs	5	Cuffed or uncuffed
6 yrs	5.5	Cuffed
8 yrs	6	Cuffed
10 yrs	6.5	Cuffed
12 yrs	7	Cuffed

Source: Reprinted with permission from D. M. Fisher.[361]

Length

Oral Tubes

Calculate the distance from the teeth or upper gum to tracheal midpoint as follows:

$$(\text{Height in cm} \times 0.1) + 5\text{ cm or}$$
$$(\text{Weight in kg} \times 0.2) + 12\text{ cm}$$

In neonates, the distance from the upper gum to the tracheal midpoint is as follows:

Weight	*Distance*
1 kg	7 cm
2 kg	8 cm
3 kg	9 cm
4 kg	10 cm

Nasal Tubes

Add approximately 20% to the oral length.

Accurate Depth Placement

The length of the trachea from the larynx to the carina is as follows:

Newborn	4 cm
6 yrs	6 cm
Adult	12–16 cm

A practical method for accurate depth placement of the tube applicable to oral and nasal intubation in pediatric patients of any size has been described as follows[159]:

- After intubation, the tracheal tube is deliberately advanced until it enters a mainstem bronchus, invariably on the right (because of the angle of the bevel), as confirmed by auscultation.
- While auscultating in the contralateral axilla, the tube is slowly retracted until breath sounds return, at which point the tube tip is at the carina. Stop retraction, and note the depth at the lips or teeth.
- The tube is retracted an additional 2 cm and secured firmly. The distal end of the tube is now safely located 2 cm above the carina.
- For children older than 6 yrs, this distance should be 3 cm.

Difficult Intubation

Intubation might be a problem in patients with the following*:

- Angioneurotic edema
- Apert's syndrome
- Carpenter's syndrome
- Cervical spine immobility
- Cherubism
- Collagen diseases
- Cri du chat syndrome
- Croup
- Cruzon's syndrome
- Cystic hygroma
- Down syndrome
- Edwards' syndrome
- Epiglottitis
- Facial trauma/burns
- Farber syndrome
- Gangrenous stomatitis
- Goldenhar's syndrome
- Hemangioma
- Klippel-Feil syndrome
- Larsen's syndrome
- Laryngeal trauma
- Meckel's syndrome
- Mucopolysaccharidoses

---

*See also Appendix D.

Myositis ossificans
Orofacial-digital syndrome
Patau's syndrome
Peritonsillar abscess
Pierre Robin syndrome
Retropharyngeal abscess
Russell-Silver syndrome
Rheumatoid diseases
Schwartz-Jampel syndrome
Scleroderma
Silver's syndrome
Smith-Lemli-Opitz syndrome
Stevens-Johnson syndrome
Treacher Collins syndrome
Turner's syndrome

Croup after Extubation

Croup after extubation manifests as a brassy cough and stertorous breathing, usually within 4 hrs after extubation but sometimes sooner in severe cases. Croup after extubation is caused by subglottic edema resulting from the following:

- A tracheal tube that is too large
- Traumatic intubation
- Coughing and bucking on the tube
- Extension and flexion of the cervical spine in the intubated patient
- Upper respiratory infection

Croup after extubation is most common in children younger than 4 yrs because of the relatively small diameter of the airway.

Management[73]

1. Add 0.5 cc of 2.25% racemic epinephrine to 4 mL saline. This mixture is placed in a micronebulizer and inhaled, assisted by positive pressure breaths, over 10–15 mins.
   Dose[307]:
      patients <20 kg: 0.25 mL
      patients 20–40 kg: 0.5 mL
      patients >40 kg: 0.75 mL
   May be repeated q1–2h.
2. Give dexamethasone, 1 mg/kg IV, and repeat q4h if needed.
3. Reintubation with a smaller tracheal tube may be necessary. Tracheostomy is rarely needed.

NOTES

NOTES

8

Ventilation

SPONTANEOUS VENTILATION

Normal respiratory rates are as follows*:

Preterm	40–60 breaths/min
Full-term	30–40 breaths/min
5 yrs	25 breaths/min
10 yrs	20 breaths/min
15 yrs	16 breaths/min

ARTERIAL BLOOD GAS TENSIONS (MM HG)

	Preterm	*Term*	*Older than 1 mo*
PaO_2[26]	60 (7.9 kPa)	70 (9.2 kPa)	95 (12.5 kPa)
$PaCO_2$[26]	37 (4.8 kPa)	39 (5.1 kPa)	40 (5.3 kPa)

Note: P_{50} of fetal hemoglobin is 19; that of adult hemoglobin is 27.
Source: Compiled from references 120, 166, 167, and 199.

Normal tidal volume at all ages is 6–8 mL/kg when breathing is spontaneous. Rate of fresh gas flow (from the anesthetic machine) is a significant factor in determining

*Modified from C. M. Mercsmar.[321]

the amount of rebreathing in the T-piece and Bain coaxial systems and thus the patient's end-expired CO_2.[6,7]

Breath-by-breath end-expired CO_2 must be monitored by a capnograph.[173] Many states require monitoring by a capnograph, and the American Society of Anesthesiologists' guidelines state, "When a tracheal tube is inserted, its correct positioning in the trachea must be verified by clinical assessment and by identification of carbon dioxide in the expired gas."[173]

Fresh gas flow should initially be 2–4 L/min and adjusted as needed. When using a circle system, there is no rebreathing of CO_2, because it is removed by the absorber. **Nevertheless, a capnograph is strongly recommended for monitoring ventilation (spontaneous or controlled) with all systems.**

WARMING AND HUMIDIFICATION OF INSPIRED GAS MIXTURES[230]

Warming and humidification of inspired gas mixtures is desirable in pediatric practice. It reduces heat and water loss in the patient, maintains ciliary activity, reduces coughing and breath holding during induction,[197] and prevents inspissation of secretions within the airways. Water content of a gas when it is fully saturated is as follows:

12.8 mL/L at 15°C (60°F)
17.5 mL/L at 20°C (68°F)
23.0 mL/L at 25°C (77°F)
30.5 mL/L at 30°C (86°F)

40.0 mL/L at 35°C (95°F)
44.0 mL/L at 37°C (98.6°F)

Inspired air has the following PaO_2 at increasing altitudes:

At sea level	149 mm Hg
At 1,000 ft	143 mm Hg
At 2,000 ft	138 mm Hg
At 3,000 ft	133 mm Hg
At 4,000 ft	127 mm Hg
At 5,000 ft	122 mm Hg
At 6,000 ft	117 mm Hg

NOTES

9

Fluid Management

COMPOSITION OF BODY FLUIDS

Source	*Sodium (mEq/L)*	*Potassium (mEq/L)*	*mOsm/L*
Bile	130	5	300
Blood	140	4.5	285–295
CSF	140	4.5	—
Diarrhea	50	35	—
Gastric	50	10–15	300
Ileum	130	15–20	300
Saliva	50	20	—
Sweat	50	5	—

Source: Reprinted with permission from W. E. Harmon.[148]

OSMOLARITY OF INTRAVENOUS FLUIDS

Fluid	*mOsm/L*
Blood	300–310
5% dextrose in water	276
Lactated Ringer's solution	276
5% dextrose in lactated Ringer's solution	552
Normal saline (0.9%)	308
5% dextrose in 0.2% normal saline	337
5% dextrose in 0.45% normal saline	410

continued

Fluid	*mOsm/L*
8.4% sodium bicarbonate	2,000
5% sodium chloride	1,760
5% albumin in lactated Ringer's solution	300 (oncotically equal to plasma)

WHAT FLUID TO USE

Most pediatric anesthesiologists use

1. D5% ¼ normal saline for maintenance fluids and for catching up on the preoperative withholding (NPO) period.
2. Lactated Ringer's solution for replacement of translocation (third space) losses.

WHAT VOLUME TO USE

The three calculations required for fluid volume management are as follows:

1. Basic hourly fluid requirements, using D5% ¼ normal saline.
2. Fluid deficit resulting from NPO, also using D5% ¼ normal saline.
3. Estimation of anticipated fluid shifts (third space) using lactated Ringer's solution.

Hourly Fluid Requirements Calculation

Volume to be given is calculated as follows:

Body weight ≤10 kg:	4 mL/kg/hr
Body weight 10–20 kg:	40 mL + 2 mL/kg/hr for each kg over 10 kg
Body weight >20 kg:	60 mL + 1 mL/kg/hr for each kg over 20 kg

For every 100 mL of water, an infant needs 3 mEq of Na^+, 2 mEq of K^+, 2 mEq of Cl, and 5 g of glucose (D5). This is provided well by D5% in ¼ normal saline and is the reason for its routine use for maintenance.[185]

Deficit Replacement Calculation

Volume to be given is calculated as follows:

1. Establish the numbers of hours from the patient's last oral intake (i.e., NPO). If the patient has been on adequate preoperative IV fluids, no deficit should exist.
2. Calculate the hourly fluid requirements as in previous section.
3. Multiply the hourly fluid requirements value by the value of NPO to determine the total deficit volume.
4. Half the volume is given in the first hour of surgery, a fourth is given in the second hour, and the remaining fourth is given in the third hour.

Fluid Shifts (Third Space or Translocation Losses)

The volume to be given is based on clinical judgment guided by information about the heart rate, diastolic blood pressure, peripheral perfusion (capillary refill, cold hands or feet), urine output (normal, 1–2 mL/kg/hr), and central venous pressure changes when available. The fluid used is lactated Ringer's solution. Provide the following:

No additional fluids for atraumatic procedures
1–2 mL/kg/hr for superficial surgery
1–2 mL/kg/hr for neurosurgery
4–7 mL/kg/hr for intrathoracic surgery
6–10 mL/kg/hr for intra-abdominal surgery

For extraperitoneal and some intraperitoneal (e.g., gastroschisis, necrotizing enterocolitis) operations, no real guidelines are available; an estimate must be made. The patient may need 10 mL/kg or more, often with added colloid (e.g., 5% albumin).

Prepyloric Losses

Replace prepyloric losses with ½ normal saline. Add K^+ (3 mEq/kg/24 hrs) if urine flow is adequate.

Postpyloric Losses

Replace postpyloric losses with lactated Ringer's solution.

Final Calculation

Intraoperative fluids given are combined as follows:

First hour:	Hourly requirements + one-half the deficit + third space losses
Second hour:	Hourly requirements + one-fourth the deficit + third space losses
Third hour:	Hourly requirements + one-fourth the deficit + third space losses
Fourth hour:	Hourly requirements + third space losses

Additional Points

1. Additional dextrose may be added to a D5% solution to make a 10% solution for premature neonates, starved neonates or infants, or infants with acute bowel pathology who are not on total parenteral nutrition. Monitor blood glucose hourly.
2. Add albumin if the total serum proteins are less than 3 g/dL.
3. If the hematocrit is very high (this may be normal for a newborn), it may be due to dehydration. If so, treat with crystalloids, or use dextran (15 mL/kg) to lower the hematocrit and reduce viscosity.
4. Sodium deficit: Using normal saline, the total amount to be replaced is calculated as follows: Na^+ deficit (mEq/L) × body weight (kg) × 0.6

   If urgent: Symptomatic hyponatremia is defined as $Na^+ <120$ mEq/L. Symptoms are lethargy, nausea, vomiting, and seizures. Use 3% saline 10 mL/kg over 5–10 mins. If necessary, repeat in 10 mins. Monitor serum sodium.

5. Potassium deficit: Replacement rate is 3–4 mEq/kg/day.[10,150] This must be given slowly. Monitor the serum K^+ and the ECG. Urine output must be adequate (0.5 mL/kg/hr).
6. Calcium infusion: Use a 2% calcium gluconate solution. Infuse at 5 mg/kg/hr.
7. Losses proximal to pylorus: Replace with ½ normal saline and add K^+ at a rate of 3 mEq/kg/24 hrs if urine flow is adequate.
8. Losses distal to pylorus: Replace with lactated Ringer's solution.

DEHYDRATION

Types

Serum type	*Osmolarity (mOsm/L)*	*Serum sodium (mmol/L)*	*Etiology*
Isotonic	270–300	130–150	Hypotonic losses (e.g., fasting, thirsting, diarrhea, vomiting) with replacement by hypotonic fluids
Hypotonic	<270	<130	Ongoing sodium loss with replacement by beverages poor in sodium
Hypertonic	>310	>150	Inadequate replacement of free water

Source: Reprinted with permission from C. Bell et al.[58]

Signs[9]

	5% (Mild)	*10% (Moderate)*	*15% (Severe)*
Sensorium	Clear	Clouded	May be stuporous
Lips and mouth	Moist	Dry	Very dry
Skin turgor	Normal	Slight reduction	Reduced
Fontanel and eyes	Normal	Slightly depressed	Sunken
Tears	Present	Dry	Very dry
Pulse rate	Normal	Tachycardia	Tachycardia
Pulse palpable	Normal	Weaker	Weaker still
Capillary refill	Normal	Normal	Sluggish/mottled
Respiratory rate	Normal	Increased	Labored
Blood pressure	Normal	Normal	Low
Urinary output	Normal	Decreased	None (anuria)
Urinary specific gravity	Normal	Raised	High

Source: Modified from S. Graves[9] and A. L. Friedman.[322]

Correction[9]

Total body water is 75–80% of body weight in neonates and 70% of body weight in infants.

Assess the degree of dehydration by using the preceding table and calculating the amount of weight loss:

Total body water × percent dehydration = volume to be replaced.

Use lactated Ringer's solution to correct isotonic dehydration.

Use D5W to correct hypertonic dehydration.

Use saline to correct hypotonic dehydration.

NOTES

NOTES

NOTES

10

Blood and Its Components

Age	*Normal hemoglobin values (g/dL)*	*Criteria for anemia (g/dL)*
Newborn	17.0–19.5	Hb <13.5 (cord blood)
2 wks	16.5	Hb <13
2 mos	14	Hb <10
6 mos	12	Hb <10
1 yr	11	—
2 yrs	11.5	—
5 yrs	12.6	—
5–10 yrs	13.1–13.5	—
>10 yrs	14.5	—

Source: Hemoglobin values extracted from A. Hackel[201] and C. Bell and Z. N. Kain.[281]

NORMAL HEMATOLOGIC VALUES DURING THE FIRST WEEK OF LIFE

Value	*Cord blood*	*Day 1*	*Day 3*	*Day 7*
Hemoglobin (g/dL)	16.8	18.4	17.8	17
Hematocrit (%)	53	58	55	54
Red cells ($\mu L \times 10^6$)	5.25	5.8	5.6	5.2
Mean corpuscular volume (μm^3)	107	108	99	98
Mean corpuscular hemoglobin (pg)	34	35	33	32.5
Mean corpuscular hemoglobin concentration (%)	31.7	32.5	33	33
Reticulocytes (%)	3–7	3–7	1–3	0–1
Nucleated red blood cells (mm^{-3})	500	200	0–5	0

Source: Reprinted with permission from D. Hatch et al.[219]

COMPOSITION

Component	*Normal whole blood in vivo*	*Citrated whole blood (at 2 wks)*	*Citrated packed cells*	*Fresh-frozen plasma*
pH	7.4	6.6–6.9	6.6–6.9	6.6–6.9
P_{CO_2} (mm Hg)	35–45	180–210	180–210	180–210
Base deficit (mmol/L)	0	9–15	9–15	9–15
K^+	3.5–5.0	18–26	18–26	4–8
Citrate	None	++++	++	++++
Factors V and VIII	Normal	20–50%	20–50%	85–100%
Fibrinogen	Normal	Normal	Normal	Normal
Platelets (per μL)	240,000–400,000	None	None	None
2,3-Diphosphoglycerate	Normal	3% normal	3% normal	—
Hematocrit (%)	35–45	35–45	60–70	—
Temperature	37°C	4°–6°C	4°–6°C	Cold

Source: Reprinted with permission from EK Motoyama, PJ Davis. Anesthesia for Trauma. In EK Motoyama, PJ Davis (eds), Anesthesia for Infants and Children (5th ed). St. Louis: Mosby, 1990.

STORED WHOLE BLOOD

- Hematocrit = approximately 40%; Na^+ = 25 mEq/L; K^+ = 15 mEq/L.
- pH varies with storage time, during which it falls (acidotic).
- 3 mL/kg raises hematocrit by 3%.[356]
- Transfusion is rarely indicated when the hemoglobin concentration is >10 g/dL and almost always when it is <6 g/dL. When values are between these, the need for

transfusion is based on the risks of complications from inadequate tissue oxygenation.[145]

*Normal Clotting Factors**

Bleeding time	209 mins
Platelet count	100,000–400,000 μ/L
Prothrombin time	10–12 secs
Activated partial thromboplastin time	25–35 secs
Fibrinogen	200–400 mg/dL
Fibrin spit products	Positive = >40 μg/mL or titer 1:50
Fibrin degradation products	Positive = >40 μg/mL or titer 1:50
D-Dimer	Positive = 1 μg/mL

COMPONENTS

Cryoprecipitate[70]

- Contains factor VIII (>100 U), fibrinogen (>150 U), factor XIII, and von Willebrand's factor.
- Average bag contains approximately 300 mg of fibrinogen in 10 mL; this is known as 1 U.
- Recommended dose for the pediatric patient is 1 U/10 kg of weight.

---

*Modified from R. C. Pascucci.[388]

- 1 U/kg raises fibrinogen by approximately 50 mg/dL.
- Indications for administration are hemophilia A, von Willebrand's disease, disseminated intravascular coagulation, and hypofibrinogenemia (e.g., congenital fibrinogen deficiencies, massive transfusions).
- Use a standard blood filter and monitor prothrombin times (normally 13–21 secs in premature neonates; 12–14 secs in older patients).

Factor VIII Concentrate

- Used for treating hemophiliacs with intraoperative hemorrhage. Load with 50 U/kg, and follow with 25–30 U q8h.
- Monitor prothrombin times (normally 13–21 secs in the premature neonate; 12–14 secs in older patients).
- Factor VIII, 1 U/kg, raises the recipient's factor VIII level by approximately 2%. Half life: 12 hrs.

Fresh-Frozen Plasma[69]

- Plasma stored for up to 25 days is acceptable.
- Volume per unit is approximately 200–250 mL.
- Needs 30–45 mins for thawing and must then be used within 6 hrs.
- Contains >70% of the procoagulants of fresh plasma.
- Dose: 10–15 mL/kg, which increases clotting factor levels by 30%, and should be enough to provide hemostasis.[145]
- Na^+ = 40 mEq/L; K^+ = 1.5 mEq/L.

- Has plasma proteins including albumin and antibodies.
- Useful in massive blood transfusion when factors V and VIII are <25% of normal.
- Monitor vital signs and ionized calcium levels when large or rapid infusions are given. Hypotension is a feature of hypocalcemia; ECG shows a widened QRS and a prolonged QT interval. Treat with $CaCl_2$, 10 mg/kg slowly IV. The rate of transfusion is limited by citrate toxicity.
- Risks include transmission of diseases, such as hepatitis (B, non-A, and non-B) and acquired immunodeficiency syndrome, and febrile and allergic reactions.

Leukocytes

- Used for treating sepsis in neonates and also for neutropenia in older children.
- Volume per unit is approximately 250 mL.
- 1 U contains 1×10^{10} white cells and a considerable amount of contaminating red blood cells.
- Graft-versus-host disease caused by transfused leukocytes can occur in any patient with immunosuppression or prolonged cytopenia. It may be prevented by using irradiated blood products.[59]

Packed Red Blood Cells

- Hematocrit = 70–80%.
- Volume is approximately 300–350 mL/U.

- Potassium content is approximately 15–20 mEq/L.
- Packed red blood cells are acidotic (pH <7.0) and low in calcium.
- If the unit being given has a hematocrit of 70–80%, 1 mL/kg increases the patient's hematocrit by 1.5%.

Platelets[156]

- Normal platelet count (per µL) is 100,000–400,000 in neonates and 150,000–400,000 in children and adolescents. Counts below these indicate thrombocytopenia.
- In general, in the perioperative period, a patient needs platelets when the count falls below 50,000/ µL and seldom when it is higher than 100,000/ µL. With counts between these levels, the risk for more bleeding is the determining factor.[145]
- 1 U of donor blood when processed yields 5.5×10.0^{10} platelets; this is called *one platelet unit*.
- 1 U/10 kg raises the count by approximately 50,000/ µL.
- Platelets may be given in the operating room to a pediatric patient whose transfused volume exceeds one blood volume or when active bleeding is present despite adequate mechanical hemostasis.[180]

Washed Red Cells

- Washed in saline.
- Hematocrit is approximately 70%, leukocytes are <10% of their original count, and plasma proteins are very diluted.

- Used when the patient has a history of nonhemolytic transfusion reaction.

BLOOD VOLUME MANAGEMENT

The current consensus risk of disease transmission by transfusion is as follows[365]:

- HIV: 1 in 676,000 transfusions
- HTLV-1: 1 in 641,000 transfusions
- Hepatitis B: 1 in 63,000 transfusions
- Hepatitis C: 1 in 103,000 transfusions

Estimation of Normal Blood Volume

Premature newborns	95 mL/kg
Term newborns	90 mL/kg
Infants	85 mL/kg
Older children	80 mL/kg
Male adolescents	75 mL/kg
Female adolescents	70 mL/kg

Alternate calculation: blood volume in mL/kg = 50 + hematocrit. Blood volume range in the premature neonate varies (60–130 mL/kg) depending on placental transfusion.

Replacement of Lost Blood[366]

- Principles of red cell transfusion for infants over age 4 mos and children are essentially the same as for adults.

- Infants have lower levels of hemoglobin at age 6 mos (9.5– 11.5 g/L), which increases to 11.5–12.5 g/L at age 2 yrs.
- Young infants rely mainly on an increase in heart rate rather than myocardial contractility to increase cardiac output in response to hypovolemia. Young infants (especially those younger than 6 mos) require more assiduous attention to volume loss and earlier volume replacement.
- Loss of up to 10% of blood volume usually does not need replacing.
- Loss of 10–20% should be assessed according to circumstances.
- Loss of 20% or more needs replacing.

Allowable Blood Loss

Allowable blood loss is calculated as follows:

$$\text{ABL} = \text{weight} \times \text{EBV} \times [(\text{Ho} - \text{Hl}) / \text{Ha}],$$

where ABL = allowable blood loss in mL/kg; EBV = estimated blood volume in mL/kg; Ha = average hematocrit, calculated by (Ho + Hl)/2; Hl = lowest acceptable hematocrit; and Ho = original hematocrit. All hematocrit values are expressed in decimal form (e.g., 0.35 for a hematocrit of 35). Usually, Hl is approximately 0.3; for neonates, it is generally 0.4.

To replace blood lost beyond the allowable blood loss, the volume of packed red blood cells needed is calculated as follows:

(Blood lost above ABL × desired hematocrit) / hematocrit of packed red blood cells

The hematocrit of packed red blood cells is approximately 0.75.

Hemodilution[134]

For intraoperative normovolemic hemodilution, the volume of blood to be removed to achieve a hematocrit of 30 is calculated as follows:

Patients estimated blood volume × [(original hematocrit – 30) / average hematocrit]

Average hematocrit is the average of the initial and minimal hematocrit (in this case 30).

Replace circulating blood volume with crystalloids (3 to 1) or colloids (1 to 1).

Hetastarch (Hespan)

- 6% hydroxyethyl starch in 0.9% NaCl injection.
- Average molecular weight is approximately 480,000.
- Each 100 mL contains the following:
  - 6 g hydroxyethyl starch
  - 0.9 g NaCl
  - 154 mEq Na
  - 154 mEq Cl
- pH (5.9) is adjusted with NaOH.
- Osmolarity is 310 mosm/L.

Advantages

- Long duration of effect.
- No risk of transmitting infectious disease.
- Low incidence of anaphylactic reactions.
- Low cost compared to albumin and plasma preparations.
- Does not interfere with normal hemostasis if the total volume infused is kept <20 mL/kg.[114]

Disadvantages

- Dilutes factor VIII and fibrinogen levels.
- Dilution prolongs activated prothrombin time and increases prothrombin time and clotting times.

ADDITIONAL INFORMATION

I. Packed red blood cells have a hematocrit of approximately 75%. Use the following to increase the patient's hematocrit:
   A. Premature neonates[11]: Give a total of ([desired % increase in hematocrit × 4] / [3 × weight in kg]) mL of packed red blood cells. This takes into account the higher blood volume per kg of weight of premature infants.
   B. Others: For each 1%, hematocrit needs to be raised as follows:
      1. Younger than 2 yrs: 1.5 mL/kg packed cells or 2.5 mL/kg whole blood.
      2. Older than 2 yrs: 1 mL/kg packed cells or 1.8 mL/kg whole blood.

II. Minor operative losses may be compensated for with lactated Ringer's solution, provided the hematocrit is not too low. Give 3 mL of lactated Ringer's solution for each 1 mL of blood lost. In neonates and infants, using lactated Ringer's solution to compensate for blood loss of more than 15% is not advisable; for blood loss less than 15%, use lactated Ringer's solution on a one-for-one basis in these patients.

III. Major losses must be replaced with packed cells or whole blood. Replace blood milliliter for milliliter, using a syringe for smaller patients. If the magnitude of the loss is in doubt, 5 mL/kg may be added to the calculation. Fresh blood (warmed and filtered) is preferable.

IV. For emergency volume replacement (e.g., when blood is not immediately available), use 5% albumin in lactated Ringer's solution; it is osmotically equivalent to plasma.

MASSIVE BLOOD TRANSFUSIONS

See Chapter 12.

TRANSFUSION REACTIONS

See Chapter 12.

NOTES

NOTES

NOTES

11

Thermal Homeostasis

MONITORING SITES

- The lower third of the esophagus is the best site for monitoring core temperature.
- Midesophageal probes may be affected by the temperature of anesthetic gases in the adjacent trachea.[160]
- Rectal temperature probes are best avoided, especially in neonates in whom fatal perforation of the rectum has occurred.

CORE TO SKIN GRADIENTS

The difference between core and skin temperature is a good indication of tissue perfusion.

Core temperature	*Skin temperature*	*Tissue perfusion*
36°C	35°C	Good
36°C	24°C	Poor
30°C	26°C	Hypothermia

THERMONEUTRAL RANGE

Thermoneutral range is the ambient temperature at which the metabolic rate, and therefore O_2 consumption, is minimal.

1-kg premature neonate	35.5°C
3-kg term neonate	33.0°C
Adult	28.0°C

THERMAL PRECAUTIONS FOR NEONATES

- Covering the patient, including the head, is the most effective way of avoiding heat loss.[158] Cover as much of the patient as possible, especially during induction, surgical preparation, and emergence.
- Insist on a heated transport incubator. Be sure the transport incubator is powered up and kept warm during the procedure.
- Warm the operating room to 24°C well in advance, to ensure that walls and equipment are warm. This practice reduces patient cooling by radiation.
- Warm the surface of the operating table with a warming blanket and an overhead heater set at 40°C before moving the patient onto it; keep this equipment in use throughout.
- Do not move the patient to the table until all preparations have been completed; leave the patient in the warmed incubator.

- Inspired anesthetic gases should be warmed and humidified. The temperature of the inspired anesthetic mixture at the patient end of the circuit should be 38°–40°C. This measure also reduces inspissation of airway secretions, making them more amenable to removal by coughing or tracheal suction. It also avoids the depression of ciliary movement caused by dry cold anesthetic gasses.
- Surgical preparation solutions must be warmed to 40°C and dried after application to prevent heat loss, which occurs if the solutions are allowed to evaporate.
- Slow-running IV solutions in pediatric patients become near room temperature by the time they reach the patient unless a special apparatus is available to keep them warm. Blood and other fluids that are to be rapidly infused should be warmed when they enter the patient's circulation.

NOTES

12

Perioperative Problems

ACIDOSIS—METABOLIC

- Sodium bicarbonate: Give 1–2 mEq/kg empirically IV. Obtain arterial blood gases and repeat at 0.3 × body weight (kg) × base deficit. For neonates, dilute the solution with an equal volume of sterile water to reduce osmolarity.
- THAM[259]: (0.3 × body weight in kg) × (base deficit in mEq) = dose in mEq of THAM IV.

AIR EMBOLISM

Indicators

- Decrease of end-expired CO_2 (P_{ETCO_2})
- Air aspirated from central venous pressure catheter
- Change in Doppler sounds
- "Mill wheel" murmur
- Tachycardia
- Dysrhythmia
- Hypotension
- Raised central venous pressure

- Cyanosis
- Q wave in lead III
- Inverted T waves in V_1–V_3

Treatment

1. Notify the surgeon, who must flood the wound with saline.
2. Discontinue N_2O and give 100% O_2.
3. Apply continuous positive pressure to the breathing circuit.
4. Compress the internal jugular veins (during cranial or facial surgery).
5. Aspirate air from central venous pressure catheter if one is in situ.
6. Turn the patient to the left lateral position.
7. Lower the entrance site to raise venous pressure there.
8. Use vasopressors for hypotension.

ANAPHYLAXIS

Substances responsible for intraoperative anaphylaxis include the following[334]:

Colloid solutions
Induction agents
Latex
Local anesthetics
Muscle relaxants
Narcotics

Latex allergy is associated with the following risk factors[333]:

- Patients with congential urogenital malformations (spina bifida) who have had several procedures and those who have been managed with urinary latex catheters, especially since birth.
- Atopy increases the risk by a factor of four.
- An allergy to tropical fruit (cross-allergy with latex).

Recognition of Anaphylaxis

- Skin flushing, urticaria, venous dilatation
- Progressive severe arterial hypotension
- Sinus tachycardia concurrent with hypotension
- Bronchospasm, which may be diagnosed in the anesthetized patient by auscultation (wheezing) or by an increase in inspired pressure (manual or ventilator)

Initial Therapy

1. Stop administration of the suspected antigen, which can be an antibiotic, a narcotic, a local anesthetic, blood or blood product, a relaxant, contrast solutions, or latex (e.g., gloves, catheters, medicines from rubber-capped bottles).
2. Maintain the airway and give 100% oxygen. Watch for early signs of laryngeal obstruction and intubate the trachea immediately.
3. Call for assistance.

4. Discontinue all anesthetic agents (if feasible).
5. Start intravascular volume expansion with crystalloid or colloid. Elevate foot of bed (Trendelenburg position).
6. Administer epinephrine ≤10 μg/kg IV; repeat if needed.

*Secondary Treatment**

1. Catecholamine infusions. Of the following, epinephrine is drug of choice:

   Epinephrine: 10 μg/kg/min IV very slowly while monitoring the effect.[262] Repeat in 20 mins prn. Infusion: 0.1–10.0 μg/kg/min.

   Norepinephrine: Begin with 0.05–1.00 μg/kg/min by infusion.[186,211] Titrate as needed up to 1–2 μg/kg/min, although more may be needed.

   Isoproterenol: 0.1 μg/kg/min by infusion, increasing slowly if needed.[250,273] Stop if tachycardia exceeds 200/min.[164] Can be given intratracheally.
2. Antihistamines: Diphenhydramine, 1–2 mg/kg IV, is the drug of choice.
3. Corticosteroids: Hydrocortisone, 1 mg/kg IV.[203] Methylprednisolone, 2–4 mg/kg IV,[324] may be the drug of choice if the reaction is suspected to be complement mediated.

---

*Modified from J. H. Levy.[215]

4. Ranitidine, 0.5–1.0 mg/kg IV.
5. Sodium bicarbonate, 1 mg/kg IV, empirically; then guided by blood gas values.
6. Albuterol, 0.15 mg/kg in 2 mL saline by nebulizer, repeated q20min if significant bronchospasm is present.
7. If the reaction is severe, an arterial line and a central venous catheter should be inserted for subsequent management.

APNEA—POSTOPERATIVE[142]

The risk of postoperative apnea within 12 hrs in the former premature infant is as follows:

- Approximately 25% if the infant is older than 44 wks postconception.
- Approximately 10% if the infant is age 60 wks postconception or younger.

Frequency and duration of apnea decreases between 1 and 20 wks postnatal age. Regional anesthesia with sedation may decrease it. Anemia increases the risk. Possible causes include the following:

Anemia
Anesthetic agents: narcotics, relaxants, sedatives
Cardiac failure
Hypocalcemia
Hyponatremia

Hypothermia
Hypoxia, hemorrhage, edema
Intracranial pathology
Low $Paco_2$
Prematurity
Sepsis

BLEEDING DURING SURGERY—EXCESSIVE

Anesthesia-Related Causes

Hypercarbia
Hypertension
Hypoxia
Resistance in the anesthetic circuit
Respiratory obstruction
Straining or coughing
Vasodilation from the anesthetic agent

Non–Anesthesia-Related Causes

Congenital anomalies
- Hemophilia
- Afibrinogenemia (rare)
- Prothrombin deficiency in newborn

Iatrogenic
- Anticoagulants
- Citrate intoxication
- Coagulopathy

- Incompatible blood transfusion
- Massive transfusion

Ineffective tourniquet
Operations on vascular tissue
Overtransfusion
Position
Systemic diseases

- Liver disease
- Platelet deficiency
- Uremia

Transfusion reactions (see Blood Transfusion—Adverse Reactions)
Venous engorgement

BLOOD TRANSFUSION—MASSIVE

The following are possible complications of massive blood transfusions:

1. Depletion of coagulation factors V and VIII. Fresh-frozen plasma, 10 mL/kg, restores them, but note that administration at a rate greater than 1.5 mL/kg/min may cause hypotension due to calcium binding by the citrate in fresh-frozen plasma. Treat this with slow IV $CaCl_2$ (10 mg/kg).[151] Monitor the ECG.
2. Depletion of platelets. Check platelet count before giving the infusion. If the count is <50,000, give 1 U/10 kg.
3. Hyperkalemia (K^+ >5.5 mEq/L) is not common. Monitor serum potassium, ionized calcium concen-

trations, and the ECG. Treat with calcium chloride 10%. The dose is 0.20–0.25 mL/kg infused *slowly* and repeated once after 10 mins if necessary.[4] Check serum ionized calcium. Treat acidosis with sodium bicarbonate and hyperventilation. Consider glucose and insulin.

4. Hypocalcemia can occur after a large transfusion of blood or fresh-frozen plasma. Hypotension is a feature. ECG shows a widened QRS and a prolonged QT interval. Treatment with calcium chloride 10% is 0.20–0.25 mL/kg infused *slowly* and repeated if necessary after 10 mins. Check serum ionized calcium.
5. Infections[365]
   HIV incidence is 1 in 676,000.
   HTLV-1 incidence is 1 in 641,000.
   Hepatitis B incidence is 1 in 63,000.
   Hepatitis C incidence is 1 in 103,000.
   Epstein-Barr syndrome, cytomegalovirus, and malaria.
6. Inability to type patient's blood: After massive transfusion, tests on post-transfusion specimens may be unreliable or frankly misleading. The best that can be done is to use blood that has been processed according to previous typing and antibody screening.[202]

BLOOD TRANSFUSION—ADVERSE REACTIONS*

Hemolytic

Signs

- Fever, flushing, hypotension, shock, tachycardia.
- Hemolysis results in free hemoglobin in serum and urine; oliguria.
- Increased bleeding (e.g., disseminated intravascular coagulation) may be the only sign in anesthetized patient.

Treatment

1. Stop the blood transfusion; keep an IV line in place.
2. Maintain good hydration to promote urine flow and support blood pressure.
3. Alkalinize the urine.
4. Centrifuge the patient's blood; check for free hemoglobin in the serum.
5. Check for hyperkalemia (K^+ >5.5 mEq/L).
6. Insert a Foley catheter, monitor urine flow, and collect a specimen.
7. Raise urinary pH with IV sodium bicarbonate.
8. Give mannitol, 1 g/kg IV.
9. Insert a central line to monitor venous pressure.
10. Send a fresh sample of the patient's blood and the bank blood to transfusion service with all details.

---

*Adapted from J. P. Scott.[318]

11. Infuse compatible packed cells to combat shock.
12. Do not use vasopressors.
13. Do not give furosemide for approximately 1 hr.
14. Watch for disseminated intravascular coagulation.

Allergic

Signs

- Tachycardia, hypotension, fever
- Urticaria, rash, periorbital edema
- Glottic edema, bronchospasm

Treatment

1. Stop the blood transfusion.
2. Administer diphenhydramine, hydrocortisone, vasopressors.
3. Treat bronchospasm if necessary.

Febrile

Signs

- Pyrexia, tachycardia, sweating, and urticaria (anaphylaxis), although blood pressure is maintained.
- Febrile reactions usually occur at the end of the transfusion.

Treatment

1. Stop the blood transfusion.
2. Administer antipyretics, diphenhydramine, and hydrocortisone. Use antibiotics if indicated.
3. Give generous amounts of fluids to maintain renal function.

BRADYCARDIA

1. Eliminate hypoxia as a cause.
2. If bradycardia is still present, give IV atropine, 0.01 mg/kg. An insufficient dose of atropine may cause bradycardia, so the minimum dose should be at least 0.1 mg IV total. Bradycardia may also be caused by stretching of tissues such as the pharyngeal muscles (e.g., at intubation), peritoneum, abdominal viscera, mesentery, anus, and so forth. Check the surgeon's activities.
3. In the neonate, hypovolemia may cause bradycardia. Try a bolus of lactated Ringer's solution, 10 mL/kg.
4. If poor perfusion and hypotension are present,[36] initiate CPR as described in Chapter 15. While performing CPR, give medications as follows:

    Epinephrine: 0.01 mg/kg IV or IO, or 0.1 mg/kg ET. Repeat the dose q3–5min.

    Atropine: 0.02 mg/kg. Minimum dose: 0.1 mg; maximum single dose: 0.5 mg for a child, 1.0 mg for an adolescent.

    Pacing (esophageal or external) may be considered.

DELAYED RECOVERY FROM ANESTHESIA

Eliminate the following as causes:

- Acidosis
- Alkalosis
- Anesthetic agents
- Cerebral edema
- Cerebrovascular incident
- Electrolyte disturbances (including calcium)
- Embolus (air, fat, thrombus)
- Hypercarbia
- Hyperthermia
- Hypocarbia
- Hypoglycemia
- Hypothermia
- Hypoxia
- Preoperative disease (e.g., diabetes)
- Perioperative medications
- Raised intracranial pressure
- Relaxants
- Shock

*Children's Coma Scale**

Ocular response: maximum score = 4

- 4 Pursuit
- 3 Extraocular movement intact, reactive pupils
- 2 Fixed pupils or extraocular movement impaired
- 1 Fixed pupils and extraocular movement paralyzed

Verbal response: maximum score = 3

- 3 Cries
- 2 Spontaneous respirations
- 1 Apneic

Motor response: maximum score = 4

- 4 Flexes and extends
- 3 Withdraws from painful stimuli
- 2 Hypertonic
- 1 Flaccid

Total maximum score = 11. Total minimum score = 3.

Glasgow Coma Scale

Possible scores = 3 minimum and 15 maximum.

Best motor response (possible 6 points)

- 6 Obeys commands
- 5 Localizes pain
- 4 Withdraws from pain

*Reprinted with permission from J Ghajar, RJ Hariri. Management of pediatric head injury. Pediatr Clin North Amer 1992;39:1107.

3 Abnormal flexion
2 Abnormal extension
1 Flaccidity

Best verbal response (possible 5 points)
5 Oriented
4 Confused
3 Inappropriate
2 Incomprehensible
1 None

Eye opening (possible 4 points)
4 Spontaneous opening
3 Opens to voices
2 Opens to pain
1 None

Modification for the very young[155]
5 Social smile; fixes and follows
4 Cries, but consolable
3 Persistently irritable
2 Restless, agitated
1 None

DIABETES INSIPIDUS[80]

I. Replace urinary losses with 2.5% dextrose in 0.2 normal saline.
II. Monitor the blood sugar. Minimum allowable levels are as follows:

A. Premature neonate: 20 mg/dL
B. Full-term neonate: 30 mg/dL
C. After 72 hrs: 40 mg/dL

III. Use vasopressin or desmopressin

A. Vasopressin infusion[35,80]
1. Dilute standard preparation to 2 mU/mL (mU = milliunit).
2. Start at 0.5 mU/kg/hr, increasing the dose until the urine output has decreased to less than 2 mL/kg/hr. Maximum: 10 mU/hr.
3. Reduce the infusion rate when urine specific gravity >1.01 and output has fallen to ≤1 mL/kg/hr.
4. Large doses cause marked vasoconstriction with the possibility of tissue ischemia and myocardial infarction.

B. Desmopressin (DDAVP)*
1. Has no cardiac side effects. Longer duration of action than vasopressin (11–12 hrs).
2. Nasally: 2.5–3.0 µg/day, best divided into two doses.[192]
3. For hemophilia: 0.3 µg/kg by slow IV infusion 30 mins preoperatively. Monitor urine output.[192]

---

*Comes as 15 µg/L. For children weighing >10 kg, dilute with 50 µL; for those weighing <10 kg, dilute with 10 µL.[131]

DISSEMINATED INTRAVASCULAR COAGULATION (CONSUMPTIVE COAGULOPATHY)

Precipitating Factors

- Acute respiratory distress syndromes (neonatal and adult)
- Burns
- Heat stroke
- Hypoxia/asphyxia
- Sepsis
- Transfusion reactions
- Trauma/shock

Diagnosis

Abnormal and excessive bleeding ("oozing from everywhere") during surgery. Laboratory confirmation includes the following:

- Low platelet count.
- Prolonged thrombin, prothrombin, and activated partial thromboplastin times.
- Low fibrinogen level. Normal levels are 125–300 mg/dL in the newborn and 200–400 mg/dL in infants and children.
- Raised fibrin split products.
- Raised level of D-dimer, a fibrin degradation product. Normal fibrin degradation product levels are <10 μg/mL.
- Low factor V and factor VIII levels.

Treatment[156]

1. Treat primary cause (e.g., shock, acidosis, hypoxia, sepsis).
2. If the prothrombin time is >16 secs, give fresh-frozen plasma, 10–15 mL/kg.
3. If fibrinogen is <100 mg/dL, give cryoprecipitate, 4 bags/m^2. Normal fibrinogen levels are 125–300 mg/dL in the newborn and 200–400 mg/dL in infants and children.
4. If the platelet count is <20,000/µL, give platelets, 4 U/m^2.

EPIGLOTTITIS

Differential Diagnosis of Epiglottitis and Laryngotracheobronchitis

	Laryngotracheobronchitis	*Epiglottitis*
Age	6 mos to 6 yrs	2–8 yrs
Cause	Virus (parainfluenza, respiratory syncytial virus)	Bacterial (*Haemophilus influenza* type b)
Season	Winter	Not seasonal
History	Gradual onset (2–3 days)	Acute onset (few hrs)
Symptoms	Irritability	Drooling (sore throat)
	Does not appear acutely ill	Appears acutely ill
	Stridor present	Stridor mild to absent
	Barking cough	Minimal cough
	Cyanosis usually absent	Cyanosis usually present
	Fever variable	High fever
	Hoarse voice	Muffled voice
	No position preferred	Prefers to be upright, chin forward
	?Retractions mild	Retractions marked
		Anxiety
X-ray findings	Subglottic narrowing	Swollen epiglottis (thumb sign)

Source: Reprinted with permission from E. D. Allen and K. S. McCoy,[232] with additions from C. Bell and Z. N. Kain.[252]

Anesthetic Management

- Do not upset the patient.
- Allow the patient to assume the most comfortable position; do not force the patient to do otherwise. Have a parent present at all times, even during the early stage of induction, to pacify and reassure the child.

- Have an otorhinologic (ear, nose, and throat) surgeon present and scrubbed and a tracheotomy tray open.
- Induce anesthesia in the operating room, using the selected agent (e.g., halothane, sevoflurane) in oxygen. The child is usually in the sitting position (toddlers do well on the parent's lap). Maintain spontaneous breathing. The parent leaves as soon as the child loses consciousness.
- Place monitors, insert an IV line, and administer atropine.
- As anesthesia deepens, assisting ventilation with gentle positive pressure may be possible.
- When the child reaches stage 3 (Geudel's signs), perform laryngoscopy and oral intubation using a stiletted tube one size smaller than would normally be used, but have a range of sizes readily available.
- When in control of the airway, change to a nasotracheal tube. Succinylcholine may be used to facilitate this change if the anesthesiologist is confident of his or her ability to visualize the larynx. A small leak around the tube should be present after intubation.
- Diagnosis can now be confirmed by visual inspection and a culture obtained from the surface of the epiglottis.

HYPERKALEMIA[55]

Causes

Accidental potassium overdose
Angiotensin-converting enzyme inhibitors, especially with decreased renal function
Infusion of triple-strength plasma
Massive transfusion with outdated blood
Muscle disease
Renal failure
Succinylcholine

In anesthesia, succinylcholine is the most common cause of a rapid rise in serum potassium. Normally, it may cause an increase of approximately 1 mEq/L, but in the following circumstances it can result in a rapid rise, from which cardiac arrest may follow, especially after a second dose of succinylcholine:

- Burn patients for the first 2–3 mos
- Patients who have been bedridden for as little as a few days but usually longer.
- Major trauma
- Paraplegia
- Cerebrovascular accidents
- Muscular dystrophies
- Uremia
- Tetanus

Diagnosis

Serum K^+ above 5.5 mEq/L. Arrhythmias start to occur at around 7.0 mEq/L, depending on the rate of increase. The following ECG changes occur sequentially:

- Tall, narrow, peaked T waves.
- P waves decrease in amplitude, widen, and then may disappear.
- R waves diminish in amplitude.
- S waves deepen.
- QT intervals widen, especially at K^+ levels >6.7 mEq/L.
- Biphasic QRST.
- Asystole or ventricular fibrillation.

Treatment

If the patient is on digitalis, a too rapid reduction in serum K^+ may unmask digitalis toxicity. Preoperative treatment comprises cation exchange resins (peritoneal or hemodialysis). More immediate treatment includes the following:

1. Hyperventilate with 100% oxygen to induce alkalosis.
2. Monitor ECG continuously.
3. Give 10% $CaCl_2$ 0.1–0.2 mL/kg slowly; this usually restores myocardial excitability in about 2 mins. Effect lasts 20 mins.
4. Sodium bicarbonate, 1–2 mg/kg IV, if a metabolic acidosis occurs. Effect peaks in 5 mins and lasts 20 mins.

5. Dextrose and insulin: Add 5 U of crystalline insulin to 20 mL D50W. Give 1 mL/kg IV over 30 mins.[171] (This may take a little time to prepare in most operating rooms.)

HYPOCHLOREMIA

Hypochloremia is a feature of pyloric stenosis, as are hypokalemia and metabolic alkalosis. Do not use lactated Ringer's solution for correction (the lactate is metabolized to bicarbonate). Infuse normal saline with additional potassium.

HYPOGLYCEMIA

Normal blood glucose levels are as follows[246]:

Premature neonate	<20 mg/dL
Full-term neonate	<30 mg/dL
After 72 hrs	<40 mg/dL

Diagnosis

Watch for hypoglycemia in the neonate who

- Is from a diabetic mother.
- Has experienced asphyxia.
- Is small for gestational age.
- Is premature.
- Has Beckwith-Wiedemann syndrome.

Signs include lethargy in the conscious patient, hypotonus, seizures, acidosis, and hypothermia. Diagnosis is confirmed by laboratory values as noted earlier.

Treatment

1. For an urgent immediate push, give dextrose 10%, 1–2 mL/kg.
2. If not urgent, give a slow IV push of D10W, 5 mL/kg (500 mg/kg) over 10 mins.[162]
3. Follow with an infusion of D10W at 2.5–5.0 mL/kg/hr.
4. Monitor blood sugar levels hourly.
5. Taper the infusion slowly after 24 hrs to avoid rebound hypoglycemia.
6. Maintain blood glucose levels between 45 and 90 mg/dL.
7. Avoid hyperglycemia: It may cause CNS damage, especially in premature neonates.

Insulin Preparations

Type	*Appearance*	*Action*	*Onset of action*	*Maximum effect*	*End of effect*
Regular	Clear solution	Rapid	0.5 hr	2–4 hrs	6–8 hrs
Neutral protamine Hagedorn isophane	Cloudy	Intermediate	1–2 hrs	6–12 hrs	18–24 hrs
Lente	Cloudy	Intermediate	1–3 hrs	6–12 hrs	18–24 hrs
Ultralente	Cloudy	Prolonged	4–6 hrs	18–20 hrs	24–28 hrs

Note: Times of onset, maximum, and duration of effect vary greatly within and between patients and are affected by many factors, including dose, injection site, exercise of the injected area, temperature, and insulin antibodies.
Source: Reprinted with permission from J. I. Wolsdorf and L. Muglia.[157]

HYPOKALEMIA[55]

The minimum safe serum concentration at which routine and emergency anesthesia may be undertaken is generally agreed to be 3.5 mEq/L. Clinical effects usually appear when the serum potassium falls below this level. However, some evidence suggests reducing this to 2.5 mEq/L. Much depends on the rate at which the lower level has occurred. Acute changes (as may occur intraoperatively) are much more hazardous. The following conditions may be observed:

- Tachycardia followed by ectopic beats
- Hypotension
- ECG:
  - T waves flattened
  - U waves present
  - QTc interval prolonged[238]

Potassium must be replaced slowly. The recommended maximum rate is 4 mEq/kg/24 hrs,[150] during which (it could take a few days) urine output must be reasonable (0.5 mL/kg/hr). Monitor serum potassium and the ECG closely.

HYPOMAGNESEMIA

Magnesium level of <1.5 mEq/L.
Causes muscle weakness, CNS depression, and hypokalemia.
Any arrhythmia or conduction disturbance is possible.[301]
QTc interval is prolonged.

Sometimes accompanied by calcium deficiency.
Treat with 25 mg/kg q4–6h IM of magnesium sulphate for three to four doses maximum.[163]
Use 50% solution for IM. Calcium gluconate is the antidote.

HYPOTENSION

Always check the patient (e.g., for pulse, perfusion, heart sounds) and blood pressure measurement technique before taking action. If onset is sudden, consider the following:

Acute hypovolemia
Myocardial depression and dysrhythmias
Inadequate ventilation with hypoxia
Medication (e.g., antibiotics, mannitol, vancomycin)
Allergic reactions (e.g., latex allergy)

If onset has been gradual, consider the following:

Overdose of anesthetic agents
Hypocarbia
Hypoxia
Hypovolemia
Low level of ionized calcium

INTRACRANIAL PRESSURE—RAISED

Symptoms	*Signs*
Early morning vomiting	Altered mental state
Headache	Bulging fontanel in infants
Irritability	Papilledema
Lethargy	Prominent scalp veins in infants
Visual disturbances	Sixth cranial nerve palsy

The data in this table are modified from M. J. Painter.[323]
Treatment includes the following[79]:

1. Hyperventilation to a $Paco_2$ of 25 mm Hg but not lower; elevate head.
2. Mannitol up to 1 g/kg over 15–20 mins.
3. Furosemide up to 1 mg/kg.
4. Dexamethasone, 0.5 mg/kg.
5. Acetazolamide, 8–15 mg PO.
6. Hypothermia.
7. Barbiturate-induced coma to a point of burst depression on the electroencephalogram.

INTRAOCULAR PRESSURE—RAISED[62]

Acetazolamide, 8–15 mg/kg IV, can be given. Avoid succinylcholine.

MALIGNANT HYPERTHERMIA[60]

Disorders Associated with Malignant Hyperthermia[109]

- Musculoskeletal
  - Ptosis
  - Strabismus
  - Kyphoscoliosis (idiopathic)
- Myopathies
  - Central core disease
  - King-Denborough syndrome
  - Muscular dystrophies
  - Myotonia congenita
- Other
  - Schwartz-Jampel syndrome
  - Previous malignant hyperthermia episode
  - ? Sudden infant death syndrome
- Patient features that may alert one to malignant hyperthermia
  - Recurrent dislocations
  - Club foot cryptorchidism
  - Short stature
  - Pes excavatum
  - First-degree malignant hyperthermia–susceptible relative

Diagnosis

Consider the diagnosis if, during anesthesia, one of the following is observed:

- Unexplained tachycardia
- Unexplained increase in end-tidal CO_2
- Inordinate rise in body temperature
- Generalized rigidity
- Mottled cyanosis
- Masseter spasm after succinylcholine
- Sweating

Differential Diagnosis

- Septicemia
- Thyrotoxicosis ("thyroid storm")
- Unsuspected pheochromocytoma
- Occult myopathy
- Neuroleptic malignant syndrome

Differential Diagnosis[234]

	Malignant hyperthermia	*Neuroleptic malignant syndrome*
Disorder	Muscle disorder of calcium metabolism	CNS disorder (e.g., Parkinson's, autonomic disorders, dystonia) in patients being treated with major tranquilizers; withdrawal of dopaminergics
Time of onset	Mins to hrs after triggering agent	Up to 2 mos after triggering agent
Trigger	Inhalation agents Succinylcholine	Major tranquilizers Metoclopramide Dopaminergic withdrawal
Treatment	Dantrolene	Stop major tranquilizer Resume dopaminergic agonist Bromocriptine ?Dantrolene
Duration	Up to a few hours	May last for more than 1 mo
Genetic transmission	Yes	No

Note: Neuroleptic malignant syndrome has been reported in children on antipsychotic medication. Symptoms are fever, rigidity, tachycardia, and autonomic instability.
Source: Reproduced with the kind personal permission of the compiler, R. Jaffe, M.D.

*Emergency Protocol for Malignant Hyperthermia**

Emergent consultation is available by calling 1-800-MHHYPER or 1-800-644-9737. Outside the United States, call 1-209-634-4917 and ask for *index zero*.

---

*Compiled from information available from the Malignant Hyperthermia Association of the United States and Norwich Eaton Pharmaceuticals. Some information is from the Association of Anaesthetists of Great Britain and Ireland supplement to *Anaesthesia* (1998;53:8). This section also has been reviewed by Scott Schulman, M.D., Department of Anesthesiology, Duke University, Durham, NC.

- Stop volatile anesthesia agents and surgery.
- Hyperventilate the patient's lungs with 100% oxygen (use a fresh breathing circuit as soon as possible, especially if halothane was in use).
- Give dantrolene, 2.5 mg/kg IV, and further doses of 1–2 mg/kg at approximately 45-min intervals as needed to control the clinical symptoms. After the symptoms subside, start 1–2 mg/kg q6–8h. Maximum dose: 10–20 mg/kg. The half-life of dantrolene is 7.3–9.3 hrs in children and 12.1 hrs in adults.[93]
- Simultaneously, start surface cooling the patient with cold water, and give cold saline IV and by other routes, such as PO and PR.
- Correct acidosis: 1–2 mEq sodium bicarbonate IV initially; be guided by arterial blood gases subsequently. Effect peaks in 5 mins and lasts for 20 mins.
- Correct hyperkalemia (K^+ >5.5 mEq/L) if necessary: Add 5 U of regular crystalline insulin to 20 mL D50W. Give 1 mL/kg initially, and titrate IV as needed.
- Monitor the ECG, temperature (skin and rectal), urine output, and arterial and central venous pressures.
- Maintain urine output at a minimum of 1–2 mL/kg/hr. Give furosemide, 0.5–1.0 mg/kg, if needed. The dantrolene vial contains mannitol (20 mg dantrolene contains 3 mg mannitol); additional mannitol, 0.25–0.50 g/kg, can be given. Check the first urine sample for myoglobin.
- Control dysrhythmia if it is persistent.[60] Give procainamide slowly at 15 mg/kg/min IV and repeat q5min

until the dysrhythmia is controlled, if hypotension ensues, if the QRS widens by 50%, or when a total of 15 mg/kg has been given. Beta blockers may be useful.

- Determine and follow arterial venous blood gases; pH; and serum levels of K^+, Na^+, Ca^{++}, lactate, creatine phosphokinase, serum glutamic-pyruvic transaminase, serum glutamic-oxaloacetic transaminase, lactate dehydrogenate, clotting factors, and urinary myoglobin.
- Observe the patient in an intensive care setting for 24–48 hrs.
- Monitor body temperature, because a recurrence may occur as late as 24 hrs after the initial episode.
- When the patient's condition has stabilized, continue IV dantrolene at 1 mg/kg q6–8h for at least 48 hrs or until a stable lowering of the creatinine phosphokinase has been achieved.

MYASTHENIA GRAVIS[81,103]

- Patients are sensitive to sedatives given preoperatively. Sedatives that depress respiration especially should be avoided.
- Drugs that aggravate myasthenia gravis are procainamide, quinidine, aminoglycoside antibiotics, phenytoin, chlorpromazine, lithium, and some diuretics.
- Local/regional anesthesia should be considered, but avoid ester local anesthetics.

- Patients exhibit an abnormal response to muscle relaxants, the features of which are
  - Extreme sensitivity to nondepolarizing relaxants.
  - Very variable effect of succinylcholine, usually favorable.
  - Phase II block appears very much earlier after succinylcholine.

Anticholinesterase treatment is recommended to be discontinued 12–24 hrs preoperatively if the clinical status of the patient allows, because anticholinesterases may increase the effect of succinylcholine and decrease the effect of the nondepolarizers. Patients become weak after stopping the anticholinesterase treatment and may not need any relaxants for most procedures, particularly because the inhalational agents produce more relaxation in these patients. After surgery, patients who have been given relaxants should receive neostigmine to restore muscle function. Some may require brief ventilatory support. Patients must also be closely observed postoperatively.

STRIDOR[317]

Associations

- Age: The younger the patient, the more likely stridor will occur.
- Allergic reactions with laryngeal edema.
- Laryngospasm.

- History of croup.
- Trauma

  Difficult or traumatic intubation.

  Tracheal tube that is too large.

  Change of head position while intubated. The more often this is done, the more likely is stridor after extubation.

  Prolonged intubation.

Treatment

1. 2.25% racemic epinephrine, 2–4 mL, in saline. Nebulize q30min.
2. Dexamethasone, 0.5–1.0 mg/kg IV.
3. Helium/oxygen to facilitate breathing.

TACHYCARDIA

Eliminate the following as causes:

Acidosis
Cardiac failure
Drugs: vagolytics and sympathomimetics (e.g., atropine, epinephrine)
Dysrhythmias*[360]
Fever (infection/sepsis)

---

*Paroxysmal supraventricular tachycardia is the most common dysrhythmia in children. Treatment is by vagotonic maneuvers (Valsalva, carotid sinus massage). If these fail, adenosine (q.v.) should be given, but if patient is unstable, cardioversion is preferred. Verapamil is also used, but in infants sudden cardiovascular collapse has been reported.

Hypercarbia
Hypovolemia
Hypoxia (tachycardia ↑ bradycardia)
Light anesthesia
Malignant hyperthermia

WHEEZING

The onset of perioperative wheezing may be due to the following:

- Reactive airways[321]
  - Asthma
  - Hypersensitivity reactions
- Bronchial mucosa edema
  - Infection
  - Increased pulmonary venous pressure
- Bronchial hypersecretion
  - Infection
  - Cholinergic drugs
- Mechanical
  - Migration of tracheal tube into the carina
  - Aspiration of pharyngeal contents past a tracheal tube that is too small

NOTES

NOTES

NOTES

NOTES

13

Local and Regional Anesthesia

CAVEATS

- Regardless of the concentration of the anesthetic solution (expressed as a percentage), the total milligrams of local anesthetic agent must be known to avoid toxic blood levels. It is useful to recall that
  a 0.25% solution contains 2.5 mg/mL
  a 0.50% solution contains 5 mg/mL
  a 1.00% solution contains 10 mg/mL
- Signs of neurotoxicity are (usually in the following order) numbness of tongue and around the mouth; lightheadedness; tinnitus; visual disturbances, sometimes with nystagmus; slurring of speech; irrational speech; loss of consciousness; seizures; and apnea.[143]
- Treatment for *neurotoxicity* includes the administration of thiopental (2–4 mg/kg IV) or midazolam (0.5–1.0 mg/kg IV) to control convulsions, and for *cardiotoxicity*, the application of advanced life support.
- Bretylium 5 mg/kg IV slowly[103] may be required to treat bupivacaine-induced dysrhythmias.

- Adding epinephrine to a local anesthetic solution prolongs the anesthetic's effect, depending on the site of injection. For example, the effect is much greater after subcutaneous infiltration than after intercostal, extradural, or brachial plexus block. Also, it has much less effect on the prolongation of the action of bupivacaine than on that of lidocaine.[143]
- Doses for infants, especially those younger than 3 mos, should be reduced by as much as one-half.

SEDATION BEFORE LOCAL OR REGIONAL PROCEDURES[53]

Before a procedure, select and administer one of the following:

- Fentanyl: ≤2 μg/kg IV alone or with 0.01 mg/kg midazolam. Half-life: 2.0–3.5 hrs.
- Diazepam: 0.1–0.3 mg/kg PO 1 hr before the procedure.
- Ketamine: 6 mg/kg nasally 30 mins preoperatively or 0.5–1.0 mg/kg IM.
- Methohexital: 20–30 mg/kg of a 10% solution PR.[259]
- Midazolam: 0.50–0.75 mg/kg PO or 1–2 mg/kg PR 30 mins before the procedure.
- Propofol: 0.5–1.0 mg/kg just before placing the block.

Pain on injection may be reduced by adding lidocaine, 0.2 mg/kg, and injecting into a large vein. Small veins on the dorsum of the hand should be avoided if possible. The antecubital fossa is suggested.[325] Postoperatively, one of the following may be given if additional sedation is needed:

- Ketamine: 0.5–1.0 mg/kg IV.
- Methohexital: 0.5–1.0 mg/kg IV.
- Propofol: 2–3 mg/kg followed by an infusion of 100 μg/kg/min.[129] See preceding paragraph on how to avoid pain on injection.

DOSE OF EPINEPHRINE FOR SURGICAL INFILTRATION IN ANESTHETIZED PATIENTS

- With enflurane or isoflurane: ≤30 μg/kg/dose maximum.
- With halothane and normocapnia: ≤5 μg/kg/dose maximum.
- Minimum interval between doses: 20 mins.

LOCAL ANESTHESIA

Topical Application

- Mucosa of mouth, nose, and larynx only: cocaine, 1 mg/kg.[261]
- Tracheal spray: lidocaine, 4 mg/kg, using a 4% solution.[291] However, because absorption is considerable and rapid in younger patients (akin to an IV injection), lidocaine should be avoided. If it needs to be administered, a 2% solution given in no more than two sprays should be used.[343]

- Intact skin: EMLA cream.[308] Maximum area of intact skin to be covered is as follows:
  - 100 cm^2 if body weight is <10 kg
  - 600 cm^2 if body weight is 10–20 kg
  - 2,000 cm^2 if body weight is >20 kg

  Cover well with an occlusive dressing for 1 hr; penetration of the local anesthetic is proportional to the duration of application.
- Disrupted skin:

  Skin lacerations and topical application: 0.50% tetracaine, 0.05% epinephrine, and 11.80% cocaine (TEC). Recommended dose for children: 3 mL.[154]

  Wound irrigation: Useful for postoperative analgesia (e.g., for hernia repairs). Flood wound for 2 mins with bupivacaine 0.25% (0.25 mL/kg), after the sac has been ligated. Repeat before skin closure.[152]

Subcutaneous Infiltration[291]

Bupivacaine[291]	2–3 mg/kg of a 0.25% or a 0.50% solution with or without epinephrine.
Chloroprocaine 2%	Maximum dose: 8 mg/kg without epinephrine; 8–10 mg/kg with epinephrine.[380]
Lidocaine[291]	5–7 mg/kg (0.5% solution = 5 mg/mL). Duration: 1 hr. 10 mg/kg with epinephrine.[319] Duration: 2 hrs.

Mepivacaine	7 mg/kg. Expected duration: 1.5 hrs.
Procaine 2%	7 mg/kg maximum dose. Duration: 1 hr.
Tetracaine[319]	Maximum dose: 2.0 mg/kg with or without epinephrine. Duration: 4–6 hrs.

REGIONAL ANESTHESIA

Nerve Blocks

Maximum doses are as follows[383]:

Bupivacaine	2.5 mg/kg; 3.5 mg/kg with epinephrine. Expected duration: 2–8 hrs.
Chloroprocaine 2%	8 mg/kg; 10 mg/kg with epinephrine. Expected duration: 0.5 hr.
Lidocaine	5 mg/kg; 10 mg/kg with epinephrine.[319] Expected duration: 1 hr.

The following *volumes* are suggested for peripheral nerve blocks in children:

- Axillary plexus block: 0.2–0.6 mL/kg[288]
- Interscalene brachial plexus block: 0.33 mL/kg[288]
- Femoral block: 0.5 mL/kg[288]
- Sciatic nerve block: 0.15–0.20 mL/kg[228]
- Inguinal paravascular (3 in 1) block: 0.5 mL/kg[228]

Axillary Block

Axillary blocks[45] are used for analgesia or surgery of the forearm.

- Use bupivacaine 0.25% (2.5 mg/mL) with or without 1:200,000 epinephrine.
- Recommended volume is ≤0.6 mL/kg (1.5 mg/kg).
- Pierce the skin with a 20-gauge needle.
- Use a 24-gauge, short-bevel, insulated needle. Attach it to a nerve stimulator.
- Set the rate to 1 stimulus/sec and the initial current to 2.5 mA to elicit direct muscle stimulation, which verifies correct functioning of equipment.
- Reduce the current to 1.5 mA, and enter the sheath. When the needle tip is correctly placed, a brisk motor response occurs.
- Reduce the current to 0.8 mA, and expect to see a continued motor response.
- Aspirate.
- If aspiration is negative and after a satisfactory test dose has been given, inject 0.30 mL/kg of bupivacaine 0.25% with 1:200,000 epinephrine.[21]

Femoral Nerve Block

Alone or in combination with other blocks, a femoral nerve block[384] is used for analgesia for fracture of the femur (pre- and postoperatively) and for any painful procedures involving the thigh (e.g., wound suture, painful dressings, burns).

In combination with a sciatic nerve block, it is effective for almost all operations on the lower limbs.

Because the nerve lies just lateral to the femoral artery, it can be located by palpating the artery. If the artery's pulsations are not palpable, Doppler ultrasonography can be used. Otherwise, the nerve can be located by setting the blockade monitor to maximum stimulus and running it along the inguinal ligament to elicit a twitch of the quadriceps, reducing the stimulus gradually to accurately locate the nerve.

- Advance a 22-gauge, 1.5-in. needle and a nerve stimulator at an angle of 45 degrees.
- When the needle pops through the sheath into the femoral compartment, the quadriceps muscle twitches markedly.
- Inject 1–2 mL of the anesthetic solution; if the twitching stops, the correct spot has been located.
- Inject the rest of the calculated volume.

The above recommendations are modified from L. Broadman.[384]

Inguinal and Iliohypogastric Block for Groin Procedures[19]

- Use bupivacaine 0.25% (2.5 mg/mL) with or without epinephrine and a 25-gauge needle.
- Infiltrate with 0.5 mL/kg of the solution in a fan-like manner, one finger's breadth medial to and one fin-

ger's breadth below the anterior superior iliac spine, just below the inguinal ligament, to block the ilioinguinal and the iliohypogastric nerves.
- Insert a 25-gauge needle just above the pubic tubercle and infiltrate with 0.5 mL/kg of the solution to block the genitofemoral nerve.
- No more than 10 mL should be needed, depending on patient size.
- Check for femoral nerve block before allowing postoperative ambulation.

Intravenous Regional Anesthesia (Bier Block)[20]

For intravenous regional anesthesia, use lidocaine 0.25%. A safe dose is 1.5 mg/kg (maximum: 3 mg/kg). The addition of vasoconstrictors is definitely contraindicated. Suggested volumes are as follows:

- 40 mL for adolescents.
- 30 mL at 10 yrs.
- 20 mL at 5 yrs.
- 10 mL at 1 yr.

The application of this block to the lower limb has been associated with a large number of toxic and neurologic complications. Dalens strongly advises against its use in pediatric patients.[342]

Paravascular Plexus "Three-in-One" Block[384]

Follow the procedure for femoral nerve block as described above. Before and during injection of the local anesthetic solution, apply firm digital pressure over the femoral sheath distal to the needle. This forces the solution to spread upward (cephalad) to block the obturator and lateral femoral cutaneous nerve as well as the femoral nerve.

Penile Block

Never use epinephrine for a penile or a digital block.

- Use a subcutaneous ring block with bupivacaine 0.25% and frequent aspirations.[153]
- The dorsal nerve of the penis may be blocked by injecting bupivacaine 0.25% deep to Buck's fascia at the base of the penis (at the 1:30 and 10:30 positions), giving 0.4 mL at each site in the newborn[208] and a little more in the older child. The drawback to this is that if any of the dorsal vessels are traumatized by the needle, a hematoma results.[384] For this reason, a ring block is preferred.

Sciatic Nerve Block

A sciatic nerve block[384] is useful for trauma of the leg, foot surgery, and especially club foot. In combination with a femoral nerve block, it is effective for almost all operations on the leg and foot.

- Place the patient in the lateral (Sims') position.
- Palpate and mark the greater trochanter and the ischial tuberosity.
- Draw a line between the two points. The sciatic nerve lies at the midpoint of this line.

- Insert a 22-gauge spinal needle, connected to a nerve stimulator, at the midpoint of the line until dorsiflexion or plantar flexion occurs in response to nerve stimulation.
- Confirm that the needle tip is in the correct fascial plane by injecting 1 mL of anesthetic solution, after which the flexion should stop.
- Inject 0.2 mL/kg, bearing in mind that the total dose should not exceed 2–3 mg/kg for bupivacaine or 7–10 mg/kg for lidocaine.

NOTES

NOTES

14

Epidural and Subarachnoid Analgesia and Anesthesia

The epidural space in children can be approached at the thoracic,[355] lumbar,[25] sacral,[386] and caudal[363] levels.

LEVEL OF STRUCTURES

The level of structures remains the same into adulthood.[53]

Age	*Spinal cord*	*Dural sac*
Neonate	L3	S3
Older than 1 yr	L1	S1

Although the distance from the skin to the lumbar epidural space at L3-4 has been evaluated by many, no reliable guide exists. Using the loss of resistance to saline test is best. A good working rule for children between the ages of 6 mos and 10 yrs is as follows: If the needle is further in than 1 mm/kg, withdraw it and reassess the approach.[297]

TEST DOSE

- Do not use air for a loss-of-resistance test: Venous air embolism, particularly dangerous in the presence of a patent foramen ovale, has been reported.[294]
- Do not rely on the aspiration test.
- To guard against intravascular injection, administer a test dose and wait at least 1.5 mins. The question is, "What should be used for the test?"
- Epinephrine, 0.5 μg/kg, is not a reliable indicator of intravascular injection in a patient anesthetized with halothane. If epinephrine is used, wait at least 5 mins to ensure no response occurs before injecting the anesthetic/ephedrine mixture. This test is less reliable with sevoflurane.
- Atropine, 10 μg/kg, can be injected as a test dose after placement of the needle or catheter.[293] A study with sevoflurane found an increase of ≥10 beats/min in heart rate and an increase in systolic blood pressure of ≥15 mm Hg after the administration of atropine.[339]
- Isoproterenol, 0.10 μg/kg in a halothane-anesthetized child or 0.05 μg/kg in an awake child, has been evaluated and is a reasonable alternative.[328]

CAUDAL EPIDURAL ANESTHESIA

Single-Shot Caudal Epidural Blockade

For a single-shot caudal epidural block, use a short-bevel, 22-gauge needle.

Clonidine

The addition of clonidine, 1–2 μg/kg, prolongs the duration of the block.[207,326] In one study (in which patients were premedicated with an analgesic), the quality and duration of postoperative analgesia was 16.6 hrs (mean), that of bupivacaine alone was 7.6 hrs (mean), and that of bupivacaine with epinephrine was 6.3 hrs (mean).[25]

Bupivacaine 0.25%

Bupivacaine 0.250% is commonly used,[21] but (especially in the very young or if the calculated volume is >20 mL) using 0.125% is better, as it provides good analgesia with less risk of exceeding the potentially toxic dose.[87] The volume used for procedures is as follows[21]:

- 0.5 mL/kg (lumbo-sacral level): circumcision, hypospadias, perianal area.
- 1 mL/kg (thoracic-lumbar level): inguinal/femoral hernias.
- 1.25 mL/kg (midthoracic block): umbilical hernia or orchidopexy.

The maximum dose of bupivacaine is 3 mg/kg (2 mg/kg for neonates and infants) with or without epinephrine.

The addition of 1:200,000 epinephrine increases duration, but sources differ on the amount of time; duration varies from 0 to 3 hrs. The most reasonable amount seems to be from 0.5 to 1.0 hr.

Lidocaine

Two dosage schemes are suggested for lidocaine:

1. Lidocaine 2%: Volume per segment = 0.08 mL + (0.008 × age in months for children younger than 4 yrs).[23]
2. Lidocaine 1.0–1.5% with 1:200,000 epinephrine[24]: 6–8 mg/kg.

Without epinephrine, the dose of lidocaine should not exceed 5 mg/kg.[293]

Ropivacaine

Ropivacaine 0.375% is given in a dose of 1 mL/kg.[371] It has similar duration of sensory blockade as the same concentration of bupivacaine but less motor block. Thus, it may be useful for postoperative pain management. In animal studies, it has been found to be less cardiotoxic than bupivacaine.

Sacral Intervertebral Approach

The sacral vertebrae remain unfused with distinct intervertebral spaces until age 18–30 yrs. The level of the S2-3 interspace is found using a horizontal line drawn at the level of the posterior superior iliac spines as landmarks. This approach has been found to be free of complications.[385]

Caudal Epidural Infusion

Caudal epidural infusion is used intraoperatively and for postoperative pain management.

Equipment

Equipment includes a 20-gauge Tuohy needle and a 24-gauge catheter or an 18-gauge Crawford needle and a 20-gauge catheter.[291] A caudally placed catheter can be reliably threaded cephalad as far as the thoracic region in neonates and children 2 yrs of age or younger.[297,363]

Infusion Solutions

- Bupivacaine 0.1% (1.0 mg/mL): After a loading dose of 0.8–1.0 mL/kg (0.8–1.0 mg/kg), infuse bupivacaine 0.1% with fentanyl, 1–2 μg/mL, at a rate of ≥0.4–0.5 mL/kg/hr (0.4–0.5 mg/kg/hr).[352] Neonates and infants should receive one-half these *concentrations*.[196]
- Chloroprocaine 3%: After a loading dose of 1.0–1.5 mL/kg, infuse at 1.5 mL/kg/hr.[311]

LUMBAR EPIDURAL ANESTHESIA

See caveats under Test Dose, on page 182.

Single-Shot Lumbar Epidural Blockade

Equipment

Tuohy needle: 17-, 18-, 19-, or 20-gauge, depending on the age of the child.

Glass syringe for the loss of resistance test:

- Children <10 kg: Use a 3-mL syringe
- Children >10 kg: Use a 5- or 10-mL syringe

Catheters:

- Children <10 kg: Use a 24-gauge catheter and a 20-gauge needle.
- Children >10 kg: Use a 20-gauge catheter and a 17- or 18-gauge needle.

Studies indicate that the caudal approach may be used successfully to site lumbar and thoracic catheters in neonates and infants, but that the success rate decreases markedly over the age of approximately 2 yrs. The lumbar approach seemed to be consistently unsuccessful.[297] Houck et al.,[351] however, have found that lumbar epidural catheters can be advanced to the thoracic region in many cases.

Level of Entry

Level of entry depends on the site of operation:

- At L2-3, the level to T8 can be obtained.
- At L3-4, the level to T10 can be obtained.

Use a small volume of saline (not air) to test for loss-of-resistance.

Drug

Use bupivacaine 0.25% with 1:200,000 epinephrine, but avoid epinephrine in babies and in the presence of cardiac abnormality. Recall that 0.25% = 2.5 mg/mL. Administer a test dose and wait 1.5 mins; do not rely on an aspiration test. The total initial dose is injected 3 mins after the test dose.

Dose

- Single dose: 0.08–1.00 mL/kg. Subsequent top-ups: 0.08 mL/kg.
- Continuous infusion: Start with a loading dose of 0.8–1.0 mL/kg.[22] Infuse at 0.1 mL/kg/hr for neonates and 0.15–0.20 mL/kg/hr in older children.[22,190] The rate of infusion varies with the relationship of the catheter tip to the incision. A lower rate is required if both are close.

Postoperative Top-Ups

Postoperative top-ups are usually needed at approximately 90 mins, although top-ups may not be needed until later in younger children. Some patients who have had no epinephrine may need top-ups at 70 mins. Catheters may remain in place for 2–7 days postoperatively, but this duration should be reduced with caudal catheters because of a greater risk of infection.

Lumbar Epidural Infusion

Lumbar epidural infusions[146] are used for intraoperative and postoperative pain management.

1. Administer a test dose of 0.1 mL/kg of 1% lidocaine with 1:200,000 epinephrine.
2. Determine the number of segments to be blocked in both directions (e.g., three segments up and three segments down equals six segments total).

3. Drug: bupivacaine 0.25% (2.5 mg/mL). Adding epinephrine to infusion solutions is not necessary because the duration of effect is determined by the infusion.
4. Initial dose: 0.056 mL/kg × number of segments to be blocked.[336]
5. Follow the loading dose immediately with an initial infusion rate of 0.1 mL/kg/hr.

Epidural Infusion of Local Anesthetics in Babies[326]

Adding epinephrine to the infusion solution is not necessary, because the duration of effect is determined by the infusion.

Bupivacaine 0.25%

Younger than 4 wks:
- Loading dose: 0.5 mL/kg; maximum: 1 mL/kg.
- Infusion: Less than 0.08 mL/kg/hr.

1 mo or older:
- Loading dose: 0.75–1.00 mL/kg.
- Infusion: 0.1–0.2 mL/kg/hr.

POSTOPERATIVE MANAGEMENT OF PATIENTS WITH AN EPIDURAL INFUSION

All of the following doses should be halved for infants younger than 6 mos.

Bupivacaine 0.1% is the local anesthetic[338]:

With no additive	0.3 mL/kg/hr. Maximum: 0.4 mL/kg/hr.
With fentanyl, 2 μg/mL	0.3 mL/kg/hr. Maximum: 0.4 mL/kg/hr.
With hydromorphone, 10 μg/mL	0.1 mL/kg/hr. Maximum: 0.2 mL/kg/hr.

The following guidelines are recommended[351]:

- Pain service must be available at all times.
- Record respiratory rate and quality and sedation/analgesia level every hour. A pulse oximeter may be useful to allow longer periods of sleep instead of frequent disturbances.
- Record heart rate, blood pressure, and pain scale every 4 hrs.
- Report changes in vital signs or analgesia promptly to the pain service.
- Pain service must evaluate the patient and the efficacy of treatment daily.

- In the patient who is at risk for respiratory depression, the following should be monitored and documented every 30 mins:
  - Respiratory rate and depth
  - Arterial artery oxygen saturation (Sao_2)
  - Heart rate
- If an opioid has been added, systemic sedatives should not be given concurrently.

EPIDURAL OPIOIDS FOR ANALGESIA[372]

- All patients should be monitored for respiratory depression for a period longer than the approximate duration of action of the last opiate given (morphine: 6–12 hrs; fentanyl: 1–2 hrs; hydromorphone: 4–8 hrs).
- Pulse oximetry (to ensure that Sao_2 remains higher than 94% when breathing room air) is the most sensitive monitor of hypoxia.[387] One report (on caudal epidural morphine) describes a case in which the onset of respiratory depression was delayed 3.5 hrs postoperatively.[350]
- Naloxone must be immediately available.[341] The dose is 10 μg/kg IV q5min until satisfactory respiration is achieved, followed by an infusion at 1 μg/kg/hr.
- After morphine, opioids administered by the parenteral route may be synergistic.
- The addition of opioids to local anesthetics (e.g., bupivacaine 0.25%) prevents the development of tachyphylaxis to the local anesthetic.

- Fentanyl rapidly diffuses out of the epidural space, so its analgesic effect is both systemic and spinal. After 60 mins, levels of analgesia are the same whether the drug has been given IV or epidurally.[340] Half-life: 20–30 mins.[347]
- Dilute in 3–5 mL saline depending on the patient's size.

Fentanyl	1-μg/kg bolus. Start an infusion of 0.25–0.50 μg/kg/hr.
Morphine	30–50 μg/kg in a preservative-free normal saline. No more than 30 μg/kg for a neonate or infant.[297] Prepare an epidural infusion solution containing preservative-free morphine sulfate, 50 μg/mL. Loading dose: 30 μg/kg. Infusion: 1–3 μg/kg/hr.[49]
Hydromorphone[338]	Use a solution of 10 μg/mL, and infuse at 0.1–0.2 mL/kg/hr. For infants younger than 6 mos, give one-half this dose.
Sufentanil[353]	0.75 μg/kg has a short onset of action. The cited study found a short duration of action and depressed ventilation during the first hour, necessitating close observation, but the incidence of side effects (e.g., pruritus, nausea, urinary retention) was low. Not the best of the epidural opioids.

Lumbar and thoracic epidural opiates[326]	Morphine, 25–50 μg/kg, can be given via catheters placed at the lumbar or thoracic level. Analgesia may last for 15 hrs or longer. The dose can be repeated if needed.

Side Effects of Opioids

- CNS
  - Sedation
  - Sensory depression
  - Somnolence
  - No motor or sympathetic depression
  - Dysphoria
- Respiratory depression
- Nausea or vomiting
- Pruritus
- Urinary retention

If side effects (except urinary retention) of narcotics prove troublesome, administer a naloxone infusion IV at 0.5–2.0 μg/kg/min. If titrated carefully, a naloxone infusion can reverse respiratory depression without affecting analgesia. Nalmefene is an alternate to naloxone. The dose is 0.5–1.0 μg/kg IV q6–8h prn, given slowly over at least 10 minutes.

SUGGESTED POSTOPERATIVE ORDERS FOR CHILDREN AFTER EPIDURAL OPIOIDS

1. An apnea monitor and a pulse oximeter (Sa_{O_2} to remain above 94%) for a period that approximates the duration of action of the last opiate given (morphine, 6–12 hrs; fentanyl, 1–2 hrs; hydromorphone, 4–8 hrs).
2. Be very careful about using IV or IM narcotics for 12 hrs after the last dose.
3. If sedation is required, use chloral hydrate, 30 mg/kg q8h PO (by nasogastric tube if needed) or PR. It does not provide analgesia.
4. Have naloxone at the bedside.
5. Call anesthesia service
   - if respiration is in question.
   - if additional analgesia is needed during the first 12 hrs after the caudal morphine.
   - if severe nausea and vomiting or urinary retention is present.
6. For severe depression of respiratory rate or apnea, start oxygenation and then administer naloxone, 1 μg/kg IV, q2–3min until satisfactory improvement occurs. Because the effect of the narcotic respiratory depression may outlast that of naloxone, continue to monitor it and reassess it every 2 hrs as long as narcotic respiratory depression is a possibility. If needed, naloxone may be infused at 0.5–2.0 μg/kg/min IV. Naloxone can be given ET using 2.0–2.5 times the IV dose (e.g., in an emergency if the IV is malfunctioning).

SUBARACHNOID (SPINAL) ANESTHESIA AND ANALGESIA

At birth, the spinal cord extends down to the level of L3, and the dural sac extends down to S3 or S4. By 12 mos, these reach the adult levels of L1 or L2 and S2, respectively.

Hemodynamic Stability[295]

- In children younger than 5 yrs, very little change in heart rate or blood pressure normally occurs, even without fluid loading. Therefore, a fluid preload is unnecessary in children younger than 5 yrs; the IV line can be established after the block has become effective. Try the feet first.
- Older children may have a significant fall in blood pressure, with the maximum fall occurring in approximately 25 mins. Not much change is seen in the heart rate.

Subarachnoid Anesthesia for Infants and Children

Drugs[375]

The following doses are for infants and children. For neonates, see the following section on Subarachnoid Anesthesia in Neonates and Formerly Premature Infants.

Lidocaine 5%	3 mg/kg with epinephrine. Duration: 30 mins.
Tetracaine 1%	0.4–1.0 mg/kg without epinephrine. Duration: 60 mins.

Tetracaine 1% 0.4–1.0 mg/kg with epinephrine.
Duration: 90 mins.

The extent of the block is related to the dose and volume injected. The formula for volume is as follows:

- Volume in milliliters needed to block one spinal segment is equal to one-tenth the patient's age in years (up to puberty).[374]
- In practice, 0.5–1.0 mL/kg is injected slowly. Maximum: 20 mL.[373]

Position

Use the left or right lateral position, but observe the following:

- Do not flex the head; the airway may become obstructed.
- The *legs should not be lifted* after spinal placement (e.g., to place a cautery pad). If the legs are lifted, the spinal will be very high. Rather, turn the patient on his or her side.

Needles

Dalens[373] recommends the following sizes of needles:

- Birth to 1 yr: 22 gauge, 30 mm long.
- 1–10 yrs: 20 gauge, 50 mm long.
- Older than 10 yrs: 18 or 19 gauge, 90 mm long.

The dead space of a 22-gauge pediatric spinal needle is 0.04 mL.

Choose the lowest possible interspace:

- At birth, the dural sac ends at S2-3 and the cord at L3.
- By age 1 yr, the dural sac rises to S1 and the cord to L1.
- Thus, to avoid the cord, the best space is L4-5, where the subarachnoid space is 1.0–1.5 cm deep. This depth increases to approximately 3 cm by age 10 yrs.

Subarachnoid Anesthesia for Neonates and Formerly Premature Infants

The mature neonate can be sedated with ketamine, 1–2 mg/kg. As in infants and children, fluid preload is unnecessary, because patients remain hemodynamically stable after placement of the block.[295] However, having an IV line in place is prudent.

Position

Use the left or right lateral position, but observe the same caveats outlined for infants and children.

Equipment

- The distance from the skin to the subarachnoid space in the neonate is 1.0–1.5 cm.
- Dalens[373] recommends a 22-gauge, 30-mm needle.

Procedure

Choose the lowest possible interspace in these patients:

- At birth, the dural sac ends at S2-3 and the cord at L3.
- By age 1 yr, the dural sac rises to S1 and the cord to L1.
- The best space is L4-5, where the subarachnoid space is 1.0–1.5 cm deep.

The characteristic "pop" is rarely felt; therefore, removing the stylet frequently is necessary to look for free flow of CSF.

Dose[375]

Bupivacaine 0.5%	0.1 mL/kg with or without epinephrine if weight is 2–5 kg.
	0.08 mL/kg with or without epinephrine if weight is >5 kg.
Tetracaine, 1 mg/mL	0.3–0.4 mL/kg, which rarely lasts more than 1 hr.

- If epinephrine is desired, add 0.02 mL of epinephrine (washing out the syringe with epinephrine is sufficient).
- Draw up the correct dose of local anesthetic in a 1-mL syringe.
- For a hyperbaric spinal, mix the calculated dose with an equal volume of 10% dextrose, as is done for an adult.

Time

Tetracaine with epinephrine provides 60–90 mins of anesthesia.

Assessment

Testing for the level of the block is difficult. Use a nerve stimulator, marching it from below to above. The child will move a shoulder upward when he or she feels it. The level should never be higher than T4.

Subarachnoid (Intrathecal) Opioids[326,375]

Preservative-free morphine, 30 μg/kg, administered in the subarachnoid space, usually provides 12 hrs or more of analgesia, but the incidence of biphasic respiratory depression has been reported to be as high as 25%. Using an intrathecal dose of ≥10 μg/kg of morphine is best. Experienced staff should monitor respiration meticulously, and naloxone must be readily available. Respiratory depression can be managed with a continuous infusion of naloxone without restoring pain.[337] Subarachnoid (intrathecal) opiates are useful for analgesia after cardiac surgery, spinal fusions, and abdominal surgery.[326]

NOTES

NOTES

15

Cardiopulmonary Resuscitation

APGAR SCORE FOR THE NEONATE

Sign	*Zero*	*One*	*Two*
Heart rate	No pulse	<100 beats/min	>100 beats/min
Respiratory effort	None	Irregular, slow, gasping	Regular, active, crying
Reflexes	Absent	Grimace	Vigorous, crying
Muscle tone	Limp	Some flexion of limbs	Active motion
Color	Pale, cyanotic	Cyanotic extremities	Pink all over

Note: Normal score at 1 min: 7–10; at 5 mins: 8–10.

RESUSCITATION

Notes[147]

1. Central venous drug delivery is best, followed by peripheral venous delivery. If a peripheral vein is used, a saline flush (minimum: 5 mL) should follow to move the drug centrally.
2. Intraosseus injection is considered to be equivalent in efficacy to the IV route.
3. The tracheal route can be used for atropine, epinephrine, lidocaine, and naloxone. For best absorption, dilute

the drug in a few milliliters of saline and inject it as deeply as possible via a catheter projecting beyond the end of the tracheal tube, followed by a few milliliters of saline and a few deep positive-pressure breaths.

4. Intracardiac injection is not recommended.

Ventilation and Chest Compression[5]

Age group	*Ventilation*	*Chest compression*	*Compression point*	*Ratio*
Neonates	30–40/min	120/min	Midsternum on the intermammary line	1:5
Younger than 1 yr	20/min	100/min	Midsternum just below the inter-mammary line	1:5
Older than 1 yr	15/min	100/min	Just above the xiphoid cartilage	1:5

How to Count

- Younger than 1 yr: 1, 2, 3, 4, 5, breathe . . . 1, 2, 3, 4, 5, breathe . . .
- Older than 1 yr: 1 and 2 and 3 and 4 and 5 and breathe . . . 1 and 2 and 3 and . . .

Notes

- This sequence provides a ratio of five compressions to one breath for all ages.[176]
- In the neonate, the sternum should be depressed 1.25–2.00 cm.
- Chest depressions must be interposed between ventilations.

DRUGS FOR RESUSCITATION OF NEONATES, INFANTS, AND CHILDREN[4,31]

Adenosine[4,360]	For symptomatic supraventricular tachycardia. 0.05–0.10 mg/kg IV followed immediately by a bolus of 2–3 mL of normal saline to avoid sequestration of the drug into red blood cells before it reaches the heart. May increase dose by 0.05 mg/kg q2min to a maximum of 0.30 mg/kg. In any event, do not exceed 12 mg/kg total.
Atropine[a]	10–30 μg/kg IV, IO, or ET.* Minimum dose: 0.1 mg. Maximum single doses: 0.5 mg/kg for a child and 1.0 mg for an adolescent.[4] May repeat doses q5min to a maximum total of 1 mg for a child and 2 mg for an adolescent. For symptomatic bradycardia.

*Drugs administered by the ET route should be diluted in 1–2 mL saline, instilled as deeply as possible into the tracheobronchial tree via a small catheter, if available, and followed by 2–5 mL of saline flush (depending on the size of the patient) and a few deep positive-pressure breaths. Atropine, epinephrine, lidocaine, and naloxone can be given ET in 2.0–2.5 times the usual doses.[4]

Bretylium	Dose: 5–10 mg/kg initially. Follow with a rapid IV infusion of fluids. A second dose of 10 mg/kg may be given if repeat defibrillation fails. For correcting ventricular fibrillation when lidocaine and defibrillation have failed.
Calcium chloride 10%	20 mg/kg IV slowly. Stop if bradycardia occurs. Repeat in 10 mins but check ionized Ca^{++} before giving more.[147] For low cardiac output. However, the American Heart Association no longer recommends its use for asystole or electromechanical dissociation; it suggests using it only when hyperkalemia, hypermagnesemia, hypocalcemia, or calcium-channel blocker overdose occurs.[4,147]
Calcium gluconate*	100 mg/kg IV slowly. May repeat the dose. For low cardiac output.
Defibrillation	Place one paddle over the heart apex and the other over the right upper chest. Use smaller paddles for patients <10 kg and adult paddles for patients >10 kg.

*Calcium chloride is preferred because it provides more active calcium.

Electrodes:

- 4.5-cm diameter for infants.
- 8- and 10-cm diameter for children.

For pulseless ventricular tachycardia or ventricular fibrillation:

- 2 J/kg or 2 watt-sec/kg. If needed, double current for two or three doses.
- If the patient has been on digoxin, start with the lowest available dose and increase it gradually.

For cardioversion of rapid ventricular or supraventricular rhythms:

- Adenosine may obviate the need for cardioversion.[360]
- Lidocaine, 1 mg/kg IV, reduces the risk of ventricular tachycardia; Valium may be needed for sedation.
- Synchronized cardioversion:
  - 0.5 J/kg. If tachyarrhythmia persists, double the dose. If conversion still does not occur, reconsider the diagnosis; sinus tachycardia may be present.[36]

Dextrose[4,286]	2 g/kg IV slow push, then 5–8 mg/kg/min. The concentration of the solution should not exceed 12.5% when used for neonates.
Dobutamine	5–20 μg/kg/min IV. Higher rates within this range are not usually needed.
Dopamine HCl	1–10 μg/kg/min IV (alpha effect predominates at >10 μg/kg/min). For hypotension and hypoperfusion.[280]
Epinephrine[4]	Two different concentrations of epinephrine solutions are needed for the recommended doses. A 1:1,000 solution contains 1 mg/mL, and a 1:10,000 solution contains 0.1 mg/mL. Be sure to use the appropriate concentration. For symptomatic bradycardia: 0.01 mg/kg (0.10 mL of the 1:10,000 solution) IV or IO. 0.10 mg/kg (0.10 mL of the 1:1,000 solution) ET. Both doses may be repeated q3–5min. Infusion: 0.1–1.0 μg/kg/min.[4]

For ET* administration:

Dose: 0.1 mL/kg of the 1:1,000 solution IV or IO.

Dilute with 3–5 mL saline. Follow with approximately 5 mL saline flush and a few deep positive-pressure breaths.

Neonates: use the 1:10,000 solution for ET administration.

For pulseless arrest:

Dose: 0.01 mg/kg (0.10 mL of the 1:10,000 solution) IV or IO.

If no response occurs, the subsequent doses are increased to 0.1 mg/kg (0.1 mL/kg of the 1:1000 solution). Repeat q3–5min during arrest.[4]

Doses of up to 0.2 mg/kg may be beneficial.[8]

If the condition persists, a high-dose infusion of 20 μg/kg/min may be commenced and reduced when an effective pulse has returned.[179]

---

*Drugs administered by the ET route should be diluted in 1–2 mL saline, instilled as deeply as possible into the tracheobronchial tree via a small catheter, if available, and followed by 2–5 mL of saline flush (depending on the size of the patient) and a few deep positive-pressure breaths. Atropine, epinephrine, lidocaine, and naloxone can be given ET in 2.0–2.5 times the usual doses.[4]

	For infusion: Start with 0.1–0.2 µg/kg/min. Titrate as needed. Maximum: 1 µg/kg/min. Usually, <0.3 µg/kg/min causes beta effects, and >0.3 µg/kg/min causes alpha effects.
Furosemide	1 mg/kg/dose IV.
Isoproterenol	Start an infusion at 0.1 µg/kg/min and titrate as needed. Usual effect is seen between 0.1–1.0 µg/kg/min. For bradycardia. Not recommended for maintaining cardiac output.
Lidocaine	1 mg/kg/dose IV. Infusion: 20–50 µg/kg/min. When given intratracheally, the dose is 2.0–2.5 times the IV dose.
Mannitol	0.25–0.50 g/kg IV over 15–20 mins to avoid hypotension. Maximum total: 12.5 g.
Naloxone	100 µg/kg IV for infants and children 5 yrs or younger or weighing 9 kg or less. Repeat as needed every 2–3 mins. For older children or those weighing more than 9 kg, an appropriate dose should be given and titrated to effect. Commence at 1 mg/kg. A total of 4 mg may be needed.[4]

	When given intratracheally, the dose is 2.0–2.5 times the IV dose. IM: 200 µg/kg.[286]
Nitroprusside	Start an infusion at 0.5 µg/kg/min. Titrate to ≤6 µg/kg/min for neonates, and 10 µg/kg/min for others.[259] Monitor blood pressure closely via an A-line. Be aware of thiocyanate toxicity (overdose, prolonged administration, renal insufficiency). See Chapter 5, page 75 for management.
Norepinephrine	Begin with 0.05–1.00 µg/kg/min by infusion.[186,211] Titrate as needed up to 1–2 µg/kg/min, but more may be needed.
Phenylephrine	IV: 5–20 µg/kg; IM: 0.1 mg/kg.[259] Infusion: 0.1–0.5 µg/kg/min IV. For hypotension from low systemic vascular resistance.
Phenytoin[324]	1.25 mg/kg IV over 2–3 mins as the loading dose. Repeat q5min, if necessary, to a total of 15 mg/kg. For ventricular tachycardia and dysrhythmias due to digitalis[150] or bupivacaine[136] toxicity. Monitor ECG.

Prostaglandin E_1	To maintain the patency of ductus: 0.1 μg/kg IV or intra-arterial.[279] Infusion: 0.1 μg/kg/min IV. Maximum rate of 0.4 μg/kg/min. Monitor for apnea, hypotension, and hypoglycemia, and maintain adequate intravascular volume.
Sodium bicarbonate	1–2 mEq/kg IV empirically, then do a blood gas and give 0.3 × kg × base deficit. For neonates, dilute the solution 1:1. Effect peaks in 5 mins, lasts 20 mins. Acidosis is due to hypoxic lactic acid production and CO_2 retention. Hyperventilation with 100% O_2 is therefore very important.
Volume[4]	15 mL/kg IV. Titrate as needed for volume management. Can be fresh-frozen plasma, blood, saline, lactated Ringer's solution, or 5% albumin in lactated Ringer's solution, depending on the patient's needs. If venous access is a problem, the IO route should be used. Bolus volumes of 10, 20, or 30 mL are given over 10 mins. The patient is reassessed after each bolus.

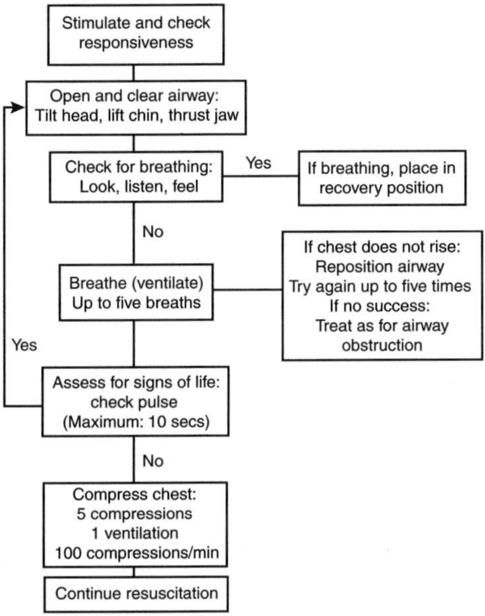

Figure 15.1. Algorithm for pediatric basic life support. (Modified from DA Zideman. Pediatric and neonatal life support. Br J Anaesth 1997;79:181; and L Chameides, MF Hazinszi [eds]. American Heart Association. Pediatric Advanced Life Support. Subcommittee on Pediatric Resuscitation, 1997;6.1–6.17.)

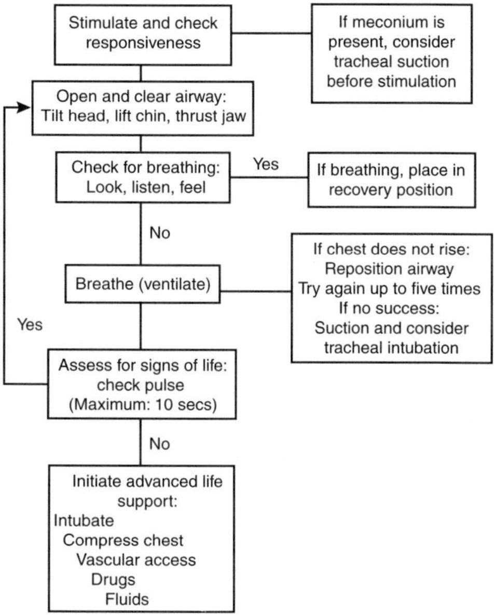

Figure 15.2. Algorithm for resuscitation of the newborn. (Modified from DA Zideman. Pediatric and neonatal life support. Br J Anaesth 1997;79:181; and L Chameides, MF Hazinszi [eds]. American Heart Association. Pediatric Advanced Life Support. Subcommittee on Pediatric Resuscitation, 1997;6.1–6.17.)

Figure 15.3. ▶Algorithm for pediatric advanced life support. (SVT = supraventricular tachycardia; VF = ventricular fibrillation; VT = ventricular tachycardia; CPR = cardiopulmonary resuscitation.) (Modified from DA Zideman. Pediatric and neonatal life support. Br J Anaesth 1997;79:181; and L Chameides, MF Hazinszi [eds]. American Heart Association. Pediatric Advanced Life Support. Subcommittee on Pediatric Resuscitation, 1997;6.1–6.17.)

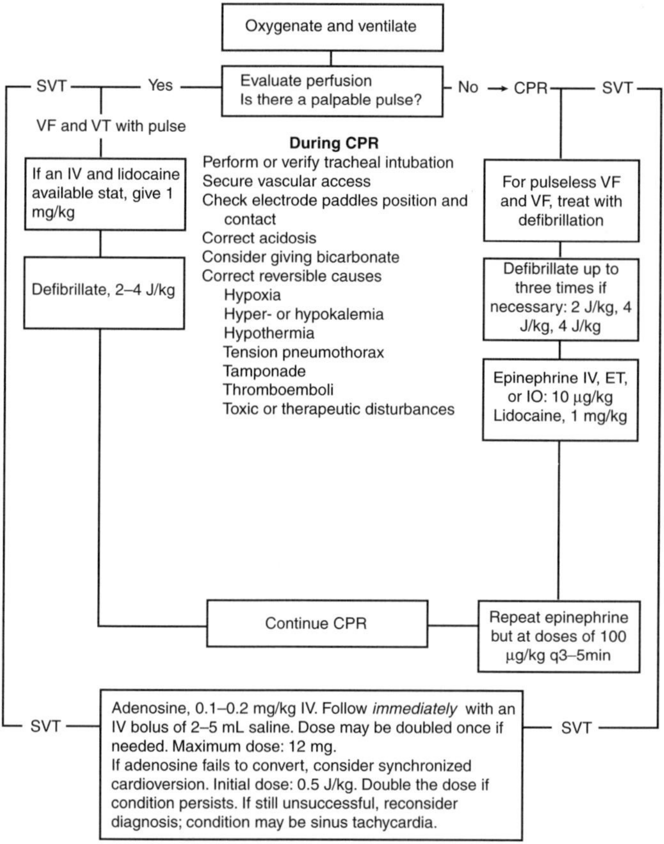
Oxygenate and ventilate
Evaluate perfusion
Is there a palpable pulse?
Yes
No → CPR
SVT
VF and VT with pulse
If an IV and lidocaine available stat, give 1 mg/kg
Defibrillate, 2–4 J/kg
During CPR
Perform or verify tracheal intubation
Secure vascular access
Check electrode paddles position and contact
Correct acidosis
Consider giving bicarbonate
Correct reversible causes
Hypoxia
Hyper- or hypokalemia
Hypothermia
Tension pneumothorax
Tamponade
Thromboemboli
Toxic or therapeutic disturbances
For pulseless VF and VF, treat with defibrillation
Defibrillate up to three times if necessary: 2 J/kg, 4 J/kg, 4 J/kg
Epinephrine IV, ET, or IO: 10 µg/kg
Lidocaine, 1 mg/kg
Continue CPR
Repeat epinephrine but at doses of 100 µg/kg q3–5min
SVT
Adenosine, 0.1–0.2 mg/kg IV. Follow *immediately* with an IV bolus of 2–5 mL saline. Dose may be doubled once if needed. Maximum dose: 12 mg.
If adenosine fails to convert, consider synchronized cardioversion. Initial dose: 0.5 J/kg. Double the dose if condition persists. If still unsuccessful, reconsider diagnosis; condition may be sinus tachycardia.
SVT

NOTES

NOTES

NOTES

Appendices

A

Normal Pediatric Values

BIOCHEMICAL VALUES

The following biochemical values are provided as a guide only. Values vary from laboratory to laboratory, because testing methods differ. The reader is advised to check each laboratory's reference range.

	Newborn	*Infant*	*Child*
Albumin (g/dL)	3.0–4.6	3.7	4.0–4.8
Base excess (mEq/L)	−4 to +3	—	—
Bicarbonate (mEq/L)	21–28	21–28	21–28
Bilirubin (mg/dL)	5–12	<16	<16
Blood urea nitrogen (mg/dL)	7–15	—	—
Calcium, ionized (mg/dL)	4.3–5.1	7.5–10.0	10
Chloride (mEq/L)	98–107	101	101
Creatinine (mg/dL)	0.3–1.0	0.2–0.4	0.3–0.7
Creatine phosphokinase (U)	<40	—	—
Fibrin degradation products (µg/mL)	<10	<10	<10
Fibrinogen (mg/dL)	125–300	200–400	200–400
Globulin (g/dL)	1.1	1.5	2.5–2.8
Glucose (mg/dL)	40–60	50–90	70–105
Hematocrit (%)	50–60	30 at 3 mos	36
Hemoglobin (g/dL)	14.5–22.5	9–14	11.5–15.5

	Newborn	*Infant*	*Child*
Magnesium (mg/dL)	1.2–2.6	1.6–2.6	1.5–2.3
Osmolarity, serum (mOsm/L)*	270–295	270–295	270–295
Partial thromboplastin time (secs)	35–50	25–35	25–35
pH	7.38–7.41	7.35–7.45	—
Potassium (mEq/L)	3.5–4.6	4–6	3.7–5.3
Protein total (g/dL)	5	5.2	5.5–7.5
Prothrombin time (secs)	13–21	12–14	12–14
Sodium (mEq/L)	133–143	133–143	133–143
Urea nitrogen (dL)	3–12	5–18	5–18
Urinary solutes (mOsm/kg/day)	10–30	—	—
Urinary Na (mEq/L)	50	—	—

Note: 1 mOsm = 19.3 mm Hg.
*Calculation: serum osmolarity = 2(Na^+ + K^+) + (blood urea nitrogen/2.8) + (glucose/18).[296] If blood urea nitrogen and glucose are normal, serum osmolarity = 2(Na^+)

Minimum values of perinatal blood glucose are as follows:

- Premature neonate: 20 dL
- Full-term neonate: 30 dL
- After 72 hrs: 40 dL

WEIGHT-MILLIEQUIVALENT VALUES[186]

	Sodium	*Potassium*	*Chloride*	*Calcium*
1 mEq equals	23 mg	39.1 mg	35.5 mg	20 mg
1 g equals	43.5 mEq	25.6 mEq	28 mEq	50 mEq
1 g NaCl has	18 mEq	—	18 mEq	—

Source: Reprinted with permission from W. E. Harmon.[148]

BLOOD

Age	*Normal hemoglobin values (g/dL)*	*Criteria for anemia (g/dL)*
At birth	19.5	Hb <13.5 (cord blood)
2 wks	16.5	Hb <13
2 mos	14	Hb <10
6 mos	12	Hb <10
1 yr	11	—
2 yrs	11.5	—
5 yrs	12.6	—

Source: Hemoglobin values extracted from A. Hackel.[201]

COAGULATION FACTORS[67,68,254]

Normal clotting requires 20% of the normal values of factor V and 30% of the normal values of factor VIII.

- Neonates (both full-term and premature):
  Prothrombin time: 13–20 secs
  Activated partial thromboplastin time: 30–55 secs
  Factors V and VIII: 100% of adult levels
  Factors IX and XI: 19% and 35% of adult levels, respectively

- Older children and adolescents:
  Prothrombin time: 10–12 secs
  Activated partial thromboplastin time: 25–35 secs
  Fibrinogen: 200–400 mg/dL
  Fibrinogen split products: <40 mg/mL

COMPOSITION OF BODY FLUIDS[148]

Source	*Na^+ (mEq/L)*	*K^+ (mEq/L)*	*mOsm/L*
Saliva	50	20	—
Gastric	60	9	300
Bile	145	5	300
Ileum	125	15	300
Diarrhea	60	30	—
Cerebrospinal fluid	140	4.5	—
Sweat	30	—	—
Blood	140	4.5	285–295

BODY SURFACE AREA[64,65]

Weight (kg)	*Body surface area (M^2)*
2	0.15
5	0.25
10	0.45
20	0.80
30	0.80
40	1.30
50	1.50

CARDIOVASCULAR SYSTEM

	Newborn	*Infant*	*Child*
Blood volume (mL/kg)	85–100*	75	70
Plasma volume (mL/kg)	50	50	50
Extracellular fluid (% body weight)	45	30	25
Intracellular fluid (% body weight)	25	40	50
Total body water (%)	80	75	65

*Blood volume range in a premature neonate is 60–130 mL/kg, depending on placental transfusion.

NORMAL HEART RATES[27]

Term	140 beats/min (range, 90–200)
6 mos	130 beats/min (range, 85–170)
1 yr	120 beats/min (range, 75–150)
7 yrs	100 beats/min (range, 70–135)
14 yrs	80 beats/min (range, 55–120)

ELECTROCARDIOGRAPHY

- P wave is due to atrial depolarization.
- Increase in amplitude is due to right atrial enlargement (lead II).
- Prolongation of the second portion is due to left atrial enlargement.
- PR interval is 0.12–0.20 sec, which represents the time required for electricity to travel from the right atrium to ventricular muscle. An increase to longer than 0.2 sec indicates a first-degree atrioventricular block. Reduction in time (conduction velocity increased)

occurs in glycogen storage disease and Wolff-Parkinson-White syndrome.

- QRS wave is due to ventricular depolarization. Duration: <0.45 sec.
- Q waves are significant if more than 2 mm deep (two small squares) or lasting longer than 0.04 sec. Higher values indicate ischemia (not necessarily recent). If the time from Q to the end of T is >0.4 sec, hypokalemia or hypocalcemia is indicated. The QT interval is also prolonged in prolonged QT syndrome.
- ST segment:
  - Depressed = ischemia
  - Elevated = acute ischemia
- T waves are normally inverted in the following:
  - Lead V_1
  - Young patients in lead V_2
  - Black patients in lead V_5
- T waves are abnormally inverted in the following:
  - After a myocardial infarct
  - V_5 and V_6 in left ventricular hypertrophy
  - V_2 and V_3 in right ventricular hypertrophy
  - Patients treated with digitalis
  - Nonspecific minor abnormalities
- A tall T wave occurs with elevated K^+ serum levels.

NORMAL CARDIAC CATHETERIZATION VALUES

	Pressure (mm Hg)	*O_2 saturation (%)*
Vena cava	—	75
Right atrium	0–3	75
Right ventricle	30/3	75
Pulmonary artery	30/10	75
Pulmonary vein	—	95
Left atrium	8	95
Left ventricle	100/8	95
Aorta	100/60	95

Source: Data from A. S. Nadas and D. C. Fyler.[161]

HEMODYNAMIC VARIABLES

Measured Values

CO Cardiac output.
Newborn: 200–250 mL/kg/min.
2 yrs: 150–200 mL/kg/min.

CVP Central venous pressure.
Mean: approximately 5 mm Hg at all ages.

RAP Right atrial pressure.
Neonate: 0–4 mm Hg.
Child: 2–6 mm Hg.[212]

LAP Left atrial pressure.
Neonate: 3–6 mm Hg.
Child: 5–10 mm Hg.[212]

MAP Mean arterial pressure.
Neonate: 65–80/45–60 mm Hg.[212]
Child: 90–110/65–75 mm Hg.[212]

MPAP Mean pulmonary artery pressure
Neonate: 65–80/35–50 mm Hg.[212]
Child: 15–25/10–16 mm Hg.[212]

C_WP Pulmonary capillary wedge pressure.
6–9 mm Hg (range, 2–14 mm Hg).

LVEDP Left ventricular end-diastolic pressure.
4–12 mm Hg at all ages.

Derived Variables

CI[165] Cardiac index = CO/m^2.
First yr of life: 2.5 $L/min/m^2$.
Age 5 yrs: 3.5 $L/min/m^2$.
Age 12 yrs: 4.25 $L/min/m^2$.

SVR[144] Systemic vascular resistance =
$[(MAP - CVP) \times 80]/CO$.
Normal:
800–1,200 dyn-sec/cm^{-5} at birth (11–18 mm Hg/L/min).
1,600 dyn-sec/cm^{-5} at 12–18 hrs (22 mm Hg/L/min).
Very little change occurs after that.

PVR[144] Pulmonary vascular resistance =
$[(MPAP - C_WP) \times 80]/CO$.
Normal: 80–240 dyn-sec/cm^{-5}
(1.5–3.0 mm Hg/L/min).

SV Stroke volume = CO/heart rate.
Normal: 50–80 mL/beat, but may be as little as 4–5 mL in neonates.

SVI Stroke volume index = SV/body surface area. Normal: 30–65 mL/beat/m^2.

QO_2 Oxygen availability = CO × arterial O_2 content.

UO_2 Oxygen consumption = CO × arterial–mixed venous O_2 difference.

CENTRAL NERVOUS SYSTEM

Parameter	*Preterm*	*Term*	*Infants and children*
Volume (mL)[52]	—	40–60	60–100
Leukocytes (cells/mL)	0–29	0–30	0–6
Protein (g/L)	0.65–1.50	0.2–1.7	0.15–0.45
Cerebrospinal fluid/ blood glucose (mg/dL)	55–105	44–248	60–90

Source: Modified from D. Hatch et al.[219]

Alternate calculations for CSF volume are as follows[63,107]:

- Children <15 kg: 4 mL/kg.
- Adults: 2 mL/kg.

By this method, a 4-kg infant has 16 mL of CSF, of which 5–7 mL lies in the spinal canal.

INTRACRANIAL BULK

CSF	11%
Blood	4%
Brain tissue	85%

CEREBRAL BLOOD FLOW[57]

Developing brain in premature neonates	30–40 mL/100 g/min
Infants and older children	65 mL/100 g/min
Adults	50 mL/100 g/min

PULMONARY SYSTEM

	Neonate	*Infant*	*Child*
Airway resistance (cm H_2O/L/sec)	30	15	2
Alveolar ventilation (mL/kg/min)	100–150	85	40
Anatomic dead space (mL/kg)	2	2	2
Closing capacity (mL/kg)	35	—	—
Closing volume	12	—	—
CO_2 production (mL/kg/min)	6	—	—
O_2 utilization (mL/kg/min)	6	8	4–5
Functional residual capacity (mL/kg)	25	30	45
Lung compliance (mL/cm H_2O)	6	20	150
Minute ventilation (mL/kg/min)	150	175	80–100
Peak flow rate (L/min)	10	—	50–450
Respiratory rate (breaths/min)	30–50	25	16
Tidal volume (mL/kg)	6	6	6
Total lung capacity (mL/kg)	63	—	—
Vital capacity (mL/kg)	40	50	60
Ratio of alveolar ventilation to functional residual capacity	4–5	—	1–2
Ratio of anatomic dead space to tidal volume	0.3	0.3	0.3
Ratio of functional residual capacity to total lung capacity	0.47	—	—
Ratio of tidal volume to functional residual capacity	0.2	0.2	0.2

ARTERIAL BLOOD GAS TENSIONS

	Preterm	*Term*	*Older than 1 mo*
$Pa{O_2}$[26] (mm Hg)	60 (7.9 kPa)	70 (9.2 kPa)	95 (12.5 kPa)
$Pa{CO_2}$[26] (mm Hg)	37 (4.8 kPa)	39 (5.1 kPa)	40 (5.3 kPa)

Note: P_{50} of fetal hemoglobin is 19; P_{50} of adult hemoglobin is 27.
Source: Compiled from references 26, 120, 166, 167, and 199.

RENAL SYSTEM

Glomerular Filtration

At birth	15 mL/min/m^2
1–2 wks	31 mL/min/m^2
0.5–1.0 yr	45 mL/min/m^2
1–3 yrs	55 mL/min/m^2
Adult	68 mL/min/m^2

Normal urine volume output should be 1–2 mL/kg/day at all ages.

NOTES

NOTES

NOTES

B

International System of Units and Other Useful Information

Important International System (SI) units in anesthesia practice include the following:

BASIC UNITS

Length	Meter (m)
Mass	Kilogram (kg)
Time	Second (sec)
Thermodynamic temperature	Kelvin (K)
Amount of substance	Mole (mol)
Electrical current	Ampere (A)

DERIVED UNITS

Frequency	Hertz (Hz): 1 Hz = 1 cycle/sec
Force	Newton (N): 1 N = 1 kg/m/sec^2
Pressure	Pascal (Pa): 1 Pa = 1 N/m^2

USEFUL EQUIVALENTS, CALCULATIONS, AND CONVERSIONS[52]

Temperature

Fahrenheit to Celsius: Subtract 32 from degrees Fahrenheit and multiply by 5/9.

Celsius to Fahrenheit: Multiply degrees Celsius by 9/5 and add 32.

Length

1 m = 39.37 in.
1 in. = 2.54 cm.
1 ft = 0.304 m = 30.480 cm.
1 yd = 0.914 m = 91.440 cm.

Mass

1 tonne (metric ton) = 1,000 kg.
1 kg = 1,000 g = 2.2 lb.
1 g = 1,000 mg.
1 mg = 1,000 μg.
1 μg = 1,000 ng.
1 mL of water at 4°C weighs 1 g.
1 L of water weighs 1 kg.
1 lb = 0.454 kg.
1 oz = 28.4 g.
1 mL of mercury (specific gravity = 13.6) weighs 13.6 g.

Volume

1 L = 1,000 mL.
1 fl oz = 29.57 mL.
1 U.S. gallon = 3.78 L.
1 Imperial gallon = 4.5 L.

Concentration

An *X*% solution contains *X* g of solute in 100 mL of solvent. For example, 5% dextrose in water contains 5 g of dextrose in 100 mL of water. A 1:1,000 solution contains 1 g of solute in 1,000 mL of solvent (e.g., water).

1:1,000 solution contains 1 mg/mL.
1:10,000 solution contains 0.1 mg/mL or 100 μg/mL.
1:100,000 solution contains 0.01 mg/mL or 10 μg/mL.
200,000 solution contains 0.005 mg/mL or 5 μg/mL.

Also keep the following in mind:

0.1% solution = 1 mg/mL.
1% solution = 10 mg/mL.
5% solution = 50 mg/mL.
10% solution = 100 mg/mL.
25% solution = 250 mg/mL.

Frequency

1 Hz is a frequency of once per sec.
50 Hz is a frequency of 50 times per sec.

0.5 Hz is a frequency of once every 2 secs.
0.1 Hz is a frequency of once every 10 secs.

Force

A newton is the force[209] that gives a mass of 1 kg an acceleration of 1 meter/sec/sec—that is, 1 N = 1 kg/s^2. The force of gravity, acting on any object, gives that object an acceleration of 9.81 meter/sec/sec. Therefore, the force of gravity acting on a mass of 1 kg is 9.81 N. This force is known as *1 kg of weight*. One Newton is equivalent to 1/9.81 kg weight, which equals 102 g of weight.

$$9.81 \text{ N} = 1 \text{ kg } (102 \times 9.81 = 1{,}000.62)$$

$$1 \text{ dyne} = 10^{-5} \text{ N}$$

Work

A joule (J) is the work done when 1 N moves its point of application 1 m in the direction of the force.

Pressure

Pressure is defined as force per unit area (e.g., lb/sq. in., N/m^2). The pascal is used throughout scientific literature, including anesthesiology texts. Because a weight of 102 g acting over 1 m^2 is very small, the kilopascal (kPa) is the most commonly used unit of pressure.[209]

$$1 \text{ Pa} = 1 \text{ N/m}^2 \text{ (also } 1 \text{ Nm}^{-2})$$

1 atm = 101.325 kPa at sea level or
= 760 mm Hg at sea level at 0°C

Therefore, 1 kPa = 7.6 mm Hg.

To convert kilopascals to millimeters of mercury, multiply by 7.6.

To convert millimeters of mercury to kilopascals, divide by 7.6.

1 kPa = 10 cm H_2O.

0.098 kPa = 1 cm H_2O.

0.133 kPa = 1 mm Hg

Conversions to International System Units

Aspirate (U/L) × 1 = U/L
Glucose (mg/dL) × 0.0555 = mmol/L
Potassium (mEq/L) × 1 = mmol/L
Serum protein (g/dL) × 10 = g/L
CSF protein (mg/dL) × 0.01 = g/L
Hemoglobin (g/dL) × 10 = g/L
White blood cells (10^3/μl) × 1 = 10^9/L
Red blood cells (10^3/μl) × 1 = 10^9/L
P_{CO_2} (mm Hg) × 0.1333 = kPa
P_{O_2} (mm Hg) × 0.1333 = kPa

These conversions are modified from B. K. Silverman.[304]

STPD Standard temperature and pressure, dry.
ST is 273.15°K or 0°C.
SP = 101.235 kPa = 760 mm Hg.

BTPS	Body temperature and pressure, saturated (assumed 37°C and 47 mm Hg).
P_b	Barometric pressure, in millimeters of mercury.
FCO_2	Fractional concentration of CO_2 in dry gas (STPD), computed as: $\%CO_2/100$.
P_{GAS}	Partial pressure, in millimeters of mercury, of a gas saturated with water vapor in the body at BTPS; assumed to be 37°C unless otherwise stated.

Conversions of 1 Standard Atmosphere (at sea level at 0°C)

1 atm = 760 mm Hg
= 101.3 kPa
= 14.69 psi
= 1.01 bar or 1,010 millibars (i.e., 1 bar = approximately 100 kPa)
= 1,000 cm or 33.96 ft of water

5,000 ft above sea level	pressure = 632 mm Hg or 84.2 kPa
10,000 ft above sea level	pressure = 500 mm Hg or 67.5 kPa
20,000 ft above sea level	pressure = 380 mm Hg or 50.6 kPa
32.8 ft below sea level	pressure = 2 atm
65.6 ft below sea level	pressure = 3 atm

Note that the pressure increase in a liquid is directly proportional to the depth.

Enough Oxygen in the Cylinder?

$$\frac{\text{Pressure in the cylinder (psi)} \times 0.28}{\text{Desired flow rate (L/min), or the time left (mins) before the supply runs out}}$$

Density

Mass per unit volume.

Energy

Energy is the capacity to do work. It uses the same unit as work (joule). One joule of work or energy (J) = the force of 1 N displaced over 1 m (1 Nm).

Power

Power is the rate of work or the rate of change of energy. Its unit is the watt (W), which equals 1 J/sec.

Osmole

An osmole is the mass of a substance that, when distributed in 22.4 L of solvent at 0°C, exerts an osmotic pressure of 1 atm. A 1-osm solution contains 1 osm/kg of solvent. Human plasma protein (60–80 g/L) exerts an osmotic pressure of approximately 25 mm Hg.

Osmolarity refers to the number of osmotically active particles per unit volume of solution (mOsm/L). *Osmolality* refers to the number of osmotically active particles per gram of water in a solution (mOsm/kg). The terms are analogous, but osmolality avoids inaccuracies from the effect of temperature on volume.

Steady State

Steady state is often incorrectly equated with equilibrium. When two components at different energy levels are brought into contact, energy flows from the higher level to the lower. If this is occurring at a steady rate, the system is said to be in a steady state. If or when the two components have the same energy level, the system will be in equilibrium.

Magnetic Field

The unit measure of the strength of a magnetic field[111] is the tesla (T).

$$1\ \text{T} = 10{,}000\ \text{gauss (G)}$$

The magnet used for MRI is in a superconductor, cooled by liquid nitrogen to 4°K, and produces up to a 2-T magnetic field. This may take 72–96 hrs to reach, so the system is never turned off, except in an emergency. Most systems operate at 1.5 T.

AD95

The AD95 is the concentration of a drug that, after equilibration, keeps 95% of patients asleep and nonreactive to surgical stimuli. AD95 values for adult patients are as follows[30]:

Halothane	0.9%
Isoflurane	1.63%
Enflurane	1.88%
Sevoflurane[112]	2.88% in children 3–5 yrs old

The AD50 is numerically identical to the MAC.[30]

Time Constant

Time constant is the time at which an exponentially changing process would have been complete had the initial rate of change been maintained.[169] In other words, it is the time in which a change from 0 to 100% would have taken place had the initial rate of change persisted (e.g., the rise of alveolar gas tension from zero toward the tension of the inspired gas).

Half-Life[56]

1. The half-life of a process is the time taken for the quantity to fall to half its initial value. At two half-lives, the substance falls to one-fourth; at three, it falls to one-eighth, and so on.

2. The elimination half-life (t½β) of a drug is the time required to clear half of the distribution volume of circulating drug. This depends on the magnitude of the distribution volume and on the activity of the metabolic clearance system.
3. See Appendix C for half-life data of selected drugs.

Compliance

Compliance is expressed as the number of units of volume change for each unit of pressure change (i.e., DV/DP). In the case of lungs, compliance is the tidal volume (the volume change) per centimeter of water (unit of pressure). The pressure referred to here is transpulmonary pressure (i.e., the difference between pleural and airway pressure).

Elastance

Elastance[138] is expressed as the number of units of pressure change for each unit of volume change (i.e., DP/DV). It is the reciprocal of compliance.

Resistance

Resistance is the pressure generated for a given flow:

$$\frac{\text{Pressure (cm } H_2O \text{ or mm Hg)}}{\text{Flow (mL/sec or L/sec)}}$$

Bohr Equation

The Bohr equation is used to calculate respiratory dead space.

$$V_D/V_T = (Paco_2 - PEco_2)/Paco_2,$$

where V_D = respiratory dead space; V_T = tidal volume; $Paco_2$ = arterial CO_2; and $PEco_2$ = mixed expired CO_2.

Laplace's Law

Laplace's law states that the difference in pressure on both sides of a spherical membrane under tension is inversely proportional to the radius of the sphere. This explains why inflating a balloon becomes easier as its size increases.

Hagen-Poiseulles Law

The Hagen-Poiseulles law describes the laminar flow of a homogeneous fluid through a rigid tube of constant length and caliber.[174] In physiology, blood is assumed to be homogeneous, and vessels are assumed to have a constant size:

$$Q = (\Delta P \pi r^4) / 8L\eta$$

where Q = blood flow (i.e., volume/time); ΔP = pressure gradient between the ends of the "tube"; r = radius of the tube (vessel); L = length of the tube (vessel); and η = viscosity of the fluid (blood).

Ohm's Law

$$I = E/R,$$

where I = amperes (current flow) = blood flow = cardiac output (Q); E = volts (force) = blood pressure; and R = resistance = vascular resistance (systemic or pulmonary).

The cardiovascular equivalent of Ohm's law may be written as Q = P/V (i.e., the flow generated is the result of the pressure applied divided by the resistance it encounters).

British Thermal Unit

The British thermal unit (BTU) is the amount of heat removed from 1 lb of water when its temperature is lowered by 1°F.

For scientific purposes, 1 BTU = 1054.8 J, which equals 252 small calories (0.25 kcal). For engineering purposes, 1 BTU = 0.293 watt hours.

Calories

Calories are the metric units of heat measurement. Written with a lower case *c*, the calorie is the amount of heat required to raise the temperature of 1 g of water from 14.5° to 15.5°C. The Calorie (with an upper case *C*) is equal to 1,000 calories and is used to express the energy value of foods. In engineering, the international calorie, which equals 1/860 watt hours, is used.

NOTES

NOTES

C

Drug Information

SERUM THERAPEUTIC RANGES

Amikacin	15–35 µg/mL.
Aminophylline	10–15 µg/L.[231]
Bretylium	0.5–1.5 µg/mL.
Bupivacaine	<4 µg/mL; higher levels are toxic.[94]
Caffeine	8–20 mg/L.
Digoxin	1.0–2.5 µg/mL; >3µg/mL may be toxic.
Dilantin	10–20 µg/mL.
Gentamicin	4–8 µg/mL.
Kanamycin	15–35 µg/mL.
Lidocaine	<6 µg/mL; higher levels are toxic.[94]
$Mg\ SO_4$	4–8 mEq/L. At 10 mEq/L, loss of deep tendon reflexes occurs.
Phenobarbital	15–40 µg/mL.
Phenytoin	10–20 µg/mL.
Procainamide	4–8 µg/mL.[172]
Quinidine	1–4 µg/mL.[172]
Streptomycin	15–35 µg/mL.
Theophylline	5–15 µg/mL.[231]
Tobramycin	4–8 µg/mL.
Vancomycin	25–40 µg/mL.

ELIMINATION HALF-LIFE OF DRUGS

The redistribution half-life of a drug ($t^{1/2}\alpha$) is the time required for the peak concentration to be reduced by 50%. For example, thiopental has a redistribution half-life of approximately 3 mins. The elimination half-life of a drug ($t^{1/2}\beta$) is the time required to clear half of the distribution volume of circulating drug. It is related to the magnitude of the distribution volume (VD) and to the activity of the metabolic clearance system as follows: $t^{1/2}\beta = [0.693 \times$ volume of distribution in a steady state $(VD_{SS})]$/clearance (Cl). The following table provides elimination half-lives of some drugs.

Acetaminophen	2–5 hrs[309]
Acetylsalicylic acid	15–20 mins[178]
Adenosine[131]	<10 secs
Alfentanil	1.5 hrs
Aminophylline	Neonate: 30 hrs[124]; child: 3–10 hrs[139]
Amrinone	Approximately 4.6 hrs
Atracurium	Infant: 20 mins; child: 17 mins; adult: 15 mins[127]
Bupivacaine	2–6 hrs[115]; younger than 6 mos: 7.7 hrs; neonate: up to 25 hrs[71] Epidural: 7.7 hrs in infants 1–6 mos; 4.6 hrs in children 5.5–10.0 yrs old
Caffeine[239]	Premature neonate: ≥30 hrs; older than 3 mos: 2–4 hrs
Chloral hydrate	Child: 25 hrs[308]
Clonidine	12–20 hrs
Cocaine	1 hr

Cortisol	8 hrs
Dantrolene	Child: 7.3–9.8 hrs[94]; adult: 12.1 hrs
Demerol[193]	3 hrs
Dexamethasone	36–54 hrs
Diazepam[239]	14–22 hrs; 25–100 hrs in neonates
Digoxin[239]	Preterm:1–2 hrs; term: 40–100 hrs; child: 28–40 hrs[303]
Diltiazem	4 hrs
Diphenhydramine	3–7 hrs
Dobutamine	Approximately 2 mins
Droperidol	101.5 ± 26.4 mins[177]
D-Tubocurarine	2 hrs[141]
Edrophonium	110 ± 34 mins[132]
Epinephrine	1.5–2.0 mins
Esmolol	10 mins
Etomidate	2–5 hrs[140]
Factor VII	5 hrs[183]
Factor VIII	8–12 hrs[183]
Factor XIII	24–60 hrs[183]
Fentanyl	2.0–4.0 hrs[308]
Flumazenil	54 mins
Gentamicin	Preterm: 3.5–16.0 hrs; term: 2.3–5.9 hrs; child: 1.2 hrs[303]
Heparin	1.0–2.5 hrs
Hydrocortisone	8 hrs
Hydromorphone	Neonate: 12–39 hrs; infant: 8–10 hrs[308]
Ibuprofen	2–4 hrs[308]
Indomethacin	Preterm:12–51 hrs; neonate: 14–20 hrs[315]

Ketamine	Younger than 3 mos: 180 mins[140]; age 4–12 mos: <65 mins; 4 yrs old: <31 mins
Ketorolac	6.1 hrs[106]
Labetalol	5–8 hrs[149]
Lidocaine	72.9 mins[85]
Lorazepam	Neonate: 40 hrs; child: 10 hrs
Meperidine	3 ± 0.5 hr; neonate: 22 hrs[314]
Methadone	12–24 hrs[347]
Methohexital	2–5 hrs[140]
Methylprednisolone	20 hrs
Metocurine	2 hrs[141]
Midazolam	1–4 hrs[308]
Morphine sulfate[100]	Newborn: 8.75 hrs; infant: 1.15 hrs; child: 0.76–1.15 hrs Epidural: 73.8 mins in children 4.5–15.0 yrs old
Naloxone	Neonate: 3 hrs; adult: 1.0–1.5 hrs[139]
Neostigmine	77 ± 47 mins[132]
Nitric oxide	3–50 secs
Ondansetron	3.5 hrs[131]
Pancuronium	2 hrs[141]
Phenobarbitone[239]	37–43 hrs; preterm: 60–200 hrs[303]
Phenytoin[71]	Neonate: 21 hrs; adult: 11–29 hrs
Physostigmine	30–60 mins
Prednisone	12–36 hrs
Procainamide	2–4 hrs
Propranolol	2–6 hrs
Propofol	1–3 hrs[140]

Pyridostigmine	12 ± 12 mins[132]
Sufentanil	Neonate: 737 ± 34.6 mins; at 12 yrs: 209 ± 23 mins
Theophylline[303]	Preterm: 12–35 hrs; child: 5–15 hrs; varies markedly
Thiopental[204]	9 ± 1.6 hrs (higher in neonates)
Vasopressin	10–20 mins
Vecuronium	70 mins[141]
Verapamil	2–5 hrs
von Willebrand factor	24–48 hrs

GENERIC NAMES OF PROPRIETARY DRUGS

Proprietary	*Generic*	*Use*
Achromycin	Tetracycline	Antibiotic
Adriamycin	Doxorubicin	Antineoplastic
Advil	Ibuprofen	Analgesic
Aldactone	Spironolactone	Diuretic
Aldomet	Methyldopa	Antihypertensive
Alupent	Metaproterenol	Bronchodilator
Amidate	Etomidate	Anesthetic
Amikin	Amikacin	Antibiotic
Amoxil	Amoxicillin	Antibiotic
Anacil-3	Acetaminophen	Analgesic
Ancef	Cefazolin	Antibiotic
Anectine	Succinylcholine	Relaxant
Antilirium	Physostigmine	Anticholinergic toxicity

Proprietary	Generic	Use
Aramine	Metaraminol	Vasopressor
Arduan	Pipecuronium	Relaxant
Aristocort	Triamcinolone	Steroid
Ativan	Lorazepam	Tranquilizer
Aventyl	Nortriptyline	Antidepressant
Bactocill	Oxacillin	Antibiotic
Benadryl	Diphenhydramine	Antihistamine
Benemid	Probenecid	Inhibits penicillin excretion
Bicillin	Penicillin G	Antibiotic
Blocadren	Timolol maleate	Beta blocker
Brethine	Terbutaline	Bronchodilator
Bretylol	Bretylium	Antidysrhythmic
Brevital	Methohexital	Anesthetic
Bricanyl	Terbutaline	Bronchodilator
Bronkodyl	Theophylline	Bronchodilator
Buprenex	Buprenorphine	Narcotic agonist-antagonist
Calan	Verapamil	Calcium blocker
Cardioquin	Quinidine	Antidysrhythmic
Cardizem	Diltiazem	Calcium blocker
Cefadyl	Cephapirin	Antibiotic
Cleocin	Clindamycin	Antibiotic
Compazine	Prochlorperazine	Antipsychotic
Corgard	Nadolol	Beta blocker
Coumadin	Warfarin	Anticoagulant
Cuprimine	Penicillamine	Inhibits penicillin excretion

Proprietary	*Generic*	*Use*
Cytomel	Liothyronine T3	Thyroid hormone
Darvon	Propoxyphene	Analgesic
DDAVP	Desmopressin	For diabetes insipidus
Decadron	Dexamethasone	Steroid
Depakene	Valproic acid	Anticonvulsant
Delta-Cortef	Prednisolone	Steroid
Deltasone	Prednisone	Steroid
Demerol	Meperidine	Narcotic
Depakene	Valproic acid	Anticonvulsant
Diamox	Acetazolamide	Diuretic
Dibenzyline	Phenoxybenzamine	Alpha blocker
Dilantin	Phenytoin	Anticonvulsant
Dilaudid	Hydromorphone	Narcotic
Diprivan	Propofol	Anesthetic
Ditropan	Oxybutynin	Antispasmodic
Dolene	Propoxyphene	Analgesic
Dolophine	Methadone	Narcotic
Dopar	Levodopa	Parkinson's disease
Dopram	Doxapram	Respiratory stimulant
Duracillin	Penicillin G	Antibiotic
Duramorph	Morphine sulfate	Narcotic
Edecrin	Ethacrynic acid	Diuretic
Elixophyllin	Aminophylline	Bronchodilator
Equanil	Meprobamate	Tranquilizer
Garamycin	Gentamicin	Antibiotic

Proprietary	Generic	Use
Halcion	Triazolam	Tranquilizer
Haldrone	Paramethasone	Steroid
Hespan	Hetastarch	Volume expander
Humatrope	Somatropin	Growth hormone
Hydeltrasol	Prednisolone	Steroid
Hyperstat	Diazoxide	Antihypertensive
Inapsine	Droperidol	Antiemetic
Inderal	Propranolol	Beta blocker
Isoptin	Verapamil	Calcium blocker
Isuprel	Isoproterenol	Beta adrenergic
Kabikinase	Streptokinase	Thrombolytic
Kantrex	Kanamycin	Antibiotic
Keflex	Cephalexin	Antibiotic
Keflin	Cephalothin	Antibiotic
Kefzol	Cefazolin	Antibiotic
Kenacort	Triamcinolone	Steroid
Kenalog	Triamcinolone	Steroid
Ketalar	Ketamine	Anesthetic
Konakion	Phytonadione	Vitamin K
Lanoxin	Digoxin	Digitalis
Larodopa	Levodopa	Parkinson's disease
Lasix	Furosemide	Diuretic
Levophed	Norepinephrine	Vasopressor
Lincocin	Lincomycin	Antibiotic
Lithane	Lithium	Antipsychotic
Lithonate	Lithium	Antipsychotic

Proprietary	*Generic*	*Use*
Lopressor	Metoprolol	Beta blocker
Marcaine	Bupivacaine	Local anesthetic
Mazicon	Flumazenil	Benzodiazapine reversal
Medrol	Methylprednisolone	Steroid
Mephyton	Phytonadione	Vitamin K
Mestinon	Pyridostigmine	For myasthenia gravis
Metaprel	Metaproterenol	Bronchodilator
Meticorten	Prednisone	Steroid
Mevacor	Lovastatin	Anti-cholesterol
Miltown	Meprobamate	Tranquilizer
Minipress	Prazosin	Antihypertensive
Mivacron	Mivacurium	Relaxant
Mycostatin	Nystatin	Antifungal
Mysoline	Primidone	Anticonvulsant
Narcan	Naloxone	Narcotic reversal
Nardil	Phenelzine	Antidepressant
Nebcin	Tobramycin	Antibiotic
Nembutal	Pentobarbital	Hypnotic
Neo-Synephrine	Phenylephrine	Vasoconstrictor/ decongestant
Nipride	Nitroprusside	Vasodilator
Norcuron	Vecuronium	Relaxant
Nuromax	Doxacurium	Relaxant
Oncovin	Vincristine	Antineoplastic
Panwarfin	Warfarin	Anticoagulant

Proprietary	*Generic*	*Use*
Pavulon	Pancuronium	Relaxant
Pen-Vee	Penicillin V	Antibiotic
Pentothal	Thiopental	Anesthetic
Pepcid	Famotidine	H_2 antagonist
Phenergan	Promethazine	Antihistamine
Pipracil	Piperacillin	Antibiotic
Pitressin	Vasopressin	Vasopressor
Procardia	Nifedipine	Calcium blocker
Proloprim	Trimethoprim	Antibiotic
Pronestyl	Procainamide	Antiarrhythmic
Prostaphlin	Oxacillin	Antibiotic
Prostigmin	Neostigmine	Reverse relaxant
Regitine	Phentolamine	Alpha blocker
Reglan	Metoclopramide	Antiemetic
Restoril	Temazepam	Sedative
Retrovir	Zidovudine	HIV therapy
Rifadin	Rifampin	Antibiotic
Rimactane	Rifampin	Antibiotic
Ritalin	Methylphenidate	CNS stimulant, antihyperkinetic
Robinul	Glycopyrrolate	Anticholinergic
Robitet	Tetracycline	Antibiotic
Seconal	Secobarbital	Hypnotic
Seldane	Terfenadine	Antihistamine
Septra	Trimethoprim	Anti-infective
Serax	Oxazepam	Tranquilizer
Solu-Cortef	Hydrocortisone	Steroid

Proprietary	*Generic*	*Use*
Stelazine	Trifluoperazine	Antipsychotic
Streptase	Streptokinase	Thrombolytic
Sudafed	Pseudoephedrine	Vasoconstrictor
Sumycin	Tetracycline	Antibiotic
Surmontil	Trimipramine	Antidepressant
Synthroid	Levothyroxine (T_4)	Thyroid hormone
Tagamet	Cimetidine	H_2 blocker
Talwin	Pentazocine	Analgesic
Temaril	Trimeprazine	Antihistaminic
Tensilon	Edrophonium	Relaxant reversal
Tetracyn	Tetracycline	Antibiotic
Tetrex	Tetracycline	Antibiotic
THAM	Tromethamine	For acidosis
Theobid	Aminophylline	Bronchodilator
Theo-Dur	Aminophylline	Bronchodilator
Thorazine	Chlorpromazine	Tranquilizer
Thytropar	Thyrotropin	Thyroid-stimulating hormone
Tigan	Trimethobenzamide	Antiemetic
Timoptic	Timolol maleate	For glaucoma
Tonocard	Tocainide	Antiarrhythmic
Toradol	Ketorolac	Analgesic
Tracrium	Atracurium	Relaxant
Trandate	Labetalol	Antihypertensive
Tridione	Trimethadione	Anticonvulsant
Trilafon	Perphenazine	Antipsychotic
Tubarine	D-Tubocurarine	Relaxant

Proprietary	*Generic*	*Use*
Tylenol	Acetaminophen	Analgesic
Unipen	Nafcillin	Antibiotic
V-cillin	Penicillin V	Antibiotic
Valium	Diazepam	Tranquilizer
Vancocin	Vancomycin	Antibiotic
Vaponefrin	Racemic epinephrine	Decongestant
Vasotec	Enalapril	ACE inhibitor
Vasoxyl	Methoxamine	Vasopressor
Velban	Vinblastine	Antineoplastic
Versed	Midazolam	Tranquilizer
Vistaril	Hydroxyzine	Tranquilizer
Wycillin	Penicillin G	Antibiotic
Xylocaine	Lidocaine	Local anesthetic
Zantac	Ranitidine	H_2 antagonist

PROPRIETARY NAMES OF GENERIC DRUGS

Generic name	*Proprietary name*
Acetaminophen	Tylenol
Acetazolamide	Diamox
Acetylcysteine	Mucomyst
Acetylsalicylic acid	Aspirin
Acyclovir	Zovirax
Adenosine	Adenocard, ATP
Adrenocorticotropic hormone (ACTH)	Acthar

Generic name	*Proprietary name*
Albuterol	Ventolin, Proventil
Alfentanil	Alfenta
Amantadine	Symmetrel
Amiodarone	Cordarone
Amikacin	Amikin
Aminocaproic acid	Amicar
Aminophylline	Mudrane, Phyllocontin
Amitriptyline	Elavil, Endep
Amoxicillin	Amoxil, Polymox
Amphotericin B	Fungizone
Ampicillin	Omnipen, Principen, Polycillin
Amrinone	Inocor
Apomorphine	Apomorphine
Atenolol	Tenormin
Atracurium	Tracrium
Beclomethasone	Beclovent, Vanceril
Betamethasone	Celestone, Uticort, Valisone
Bleomycin	Blenoxane
Bretylium	Bretylol
Bumetanide	Bumex
Bupivacaine	Marcaine, Sensorcaine
Buprenorphine	Buprenex
Butorphanol	Stadol
Captopril	Capoten
Carbamazepine	Tegretol
Carbenicillin	Geocillin
Cefaclor	Ceclor

Generic name	*Proprietary name*
Cefamandole	Mandol
Cefazolin	Ancef, Kefzol
Cefotaxime	Claforan
Cefoxitin	Mefoxin
Ceftazidime	Fortaz
Ceftriaxone	Rocephin
Cefuroxime	Ceftin
Cephalexin	Keflex
Cephalothin	Keflin
Cephapirin	Cefadyl
Chloramphenicol	Chloromycetin
Chloroprocaine	Nesacaine
Chlorothiazide	Diuril
Chlorpromazine	Thorazine
Cimetidine	Tagamet
Clindamycin	Cleocin
Clonidine	Catapres
Cortisol	Cortef, Hydrocortone, Solu-Cortef
Cortisone	Cortone
Cosyntropin	Cortrosyn
Cromolyn	Crolom, Intal, Nasalcrom
Cyclophosphamide	Cytoxan, Neosar
Cyclosporine	Sandimmune
D-Tubocurarine	Tubarine
Dantrolene	Dantrium
Desflurane	Suprane

Generic name	*Proprietary name*
Desmopressin	DDAVP, Stimate
Dexamethasone	Decadron, Hexadrol
Diazepam	Valium
Diazoxide	Hyperstat, Proglycem
Diclofenac	Cataflam, Voltaren
Digoxin	Lanoxin
Diltiazem	Cardizem, Dilacor
Diphenhydramine	Benadryl, Nytol, Sominex
Dobutamine	Dobutrex
Dopamine	Intropin
Doxacurium	Nuromax
Doxapram	Dopram
Doxorubicin	Adriamycin
Doxycycline	Vibramycin
Droperidol	Inapsine
Edrophonium	Tensilon, Reversol, Enlon
Enalapril	Vasotec
Enflurane	Ethrane
Epinephrine	Epipen
Erythromycin	E-Mycin, Ery-Tab, Ilosone, Wyamycin S
Esmolol	Brevibloc
Ethacrynic acid	Edecrin
Etodolac	Lodine
Etomidate	Amidate
Famotidine	Pepcid
Fentanyl	Sublimaze

Generic name	*Proprietary name*
Fentanyl/droperidol	Innovar
Flumazenil	Romazicon
Flurazepam	Dalmane
Furosemide	Lasix
Gentamycin	Garamycin
Glucagon	Glucagon
Glycopyrrolate	Robinul
Haloperidol	Haldol
Halothane	Fluothane
Heparin	Heparin
Hetastarch	Hespan
Hydrochlorothiazide	Esidrix, Hydrodiuril, Oretic
Hydrocortisone	Hydrocortone, Solu-Cortef
Hydromorphone	Dilaudid
Hydroxocobalamin	Cyanocobalamin
Hydroxyzine	Vistaril, Atarax
Ibuprofen	Motrin, Nuprin, Advil
Indomethacin	Indocin
Isoetharine	Bronkosol
Isoflurane	Forane
Isoproterenol	Isuprel
Kanamycin	Kantrex
Ketamine	Ketalar
Ketorolac	Toradol
Labetalol	Trandate, Normodyne
Levarterenol	Levophed
Lidocaine	Xylocaine

Generic name	*Proprietary name*
Lincomycin	Lincocin
Lorazepam	Ativan
Mannitol	Mannitol
Meperidine	Demerol
Mephentermine	Wyamine
Mepivacaine	Carbocaine, Prolocaine
Meprobamate	Equanil, Miltown, Meprospan
Metaproterenol	Alupent, Metaprel
Metaraminol	Aramine
Methadone	Dolophine
Methicillin	Staphcillin
Methohexital	Brevital
Methoxamine	Vasoxyl
Methylprednisolone	Solu-Medrol, Medrol
Metoclopramide	Reglan
Metocurine	Metubine
Metoprolol	Lopressor
Metronidazole	Flagyl, Protostat
Midazolam	Versed
Mivacurium	Nuromax
Morphine sulfate	Astramorph, Duramorph
Moxalactam	Moxam
Nafcillin	Unipen
Naloxone	Narcan
Neomycin	Neosporin
Neostigmine	Prostigmin
Nifedipine	Procardia, Adalat

Generic name	Proprietary name
Nitroprusside	Nipride
Norepinephrine	Levophed
Ondansetron	Zofran
Oxacillin	Prostaphlin
Oxytocin	Pitocin, Syntocinon
Pancuronium	Pavulon
Paromomycin	Humatin
Penicillin G	Crysticillin
Pentazocine	Talwin, Talacen
Pentobarbital	Nembutal
Pentolinium	Ansolysen
Phenobarbital	Phenobarbital
Phenoxybenzamine	Dibenzyline
Phentolamine	Regitine
Phenylephrine	Neo-Synephrine
Phenytoin	Dilantin
Physostigmine	Antilirium
Pipecuronium	Arduan
Polymixin B	Aerosporin
Prednisolone	Hydeltrasol, Pediapred
Prednisone	Deltasone, Meticorten, Sterapred
Procainamide	Pronestyl, Procan
Procaine	Novocain
Propranolol	Inderal
Pyridostigmine	Mestinon
Ranitidine	Zantac
Rocuronium	Zemuron

Generic name	*Proprietary name*
Secobarbital	Seconal
Sevoflurane	Ultane
Sodium citrate	Bicitra
Spironolactone	Aldactone
Streptomycin	Streptomycin
Succinylcholine	Anectine
Sufentanil	Sufenta
Sumatriptan	Imitrex
Temazepam	Restoril
Terbutaline	Bricanyl, Brethine
Tetracaine	Pontocaine
Tetracycline	Achromycin V, Tetrex
Thiopental	Pentothal
Timolol	Blocadren, Timoptic
Tobramycin	Nebcin, Tobrex
Tolazoline	Priscoline
Triamcinolone	Aristocort, Kenacort
Trimeprazine	Temaril
Trimethaphan	Arfonad
Trimethobenzamide	Tigan, Navogan
Trimethoprim	Septra, Bactrim
Valproic acid	Depakene
Vancomycin	Vancocin, Vancoled
Vasopressin	Pitressin
Vecuronium	Norcuron
Verapamil	Isoptin, Calan
Vitamin K_1	AquaMEPHYTON, Konakion
Warfarin	Coumadin

NOTES

NOTES

NOTES

D

Index of Syndromes and Anomalies and Their Anesthetic Implications*

Adrenogenital syndrome

Desc. Inability to synthesize hydrocortisone and possibly aldosterone; virilization of female

Impl. All patients need hydrocortisone even if not salt-losing; check electrolytes

Albers-Schönberg disease (marble bone disease or osteopetrosis)

Desc. Brittle bones, pathologic fractures

Impl. Anemia from marrow sclerosis; hepatosplenomegaly; care in positioning and restraint; limited joint mobility

*Source: Adapted from AEP Jones, DA Pelton. An index of syndromes and their anaesthetic implications. Can Anaesth Soc J 1976;23:207–223; with additions from references 191, 240, 241, and 290.

Albright-Butler syndrome

Desc. Renal tubular acidosis; hypokalemia; renal calculi

Impl. Correct electrolytes to within normal limits; renal impairment

Albright's hereditary osteodystrophy (pseudohypoparathyroidism)

Desc. Ectopic bone formation; mental retardation

Impl. Hypocalcemia: possible ECG conduction defects and neuromuscular problems; convulsions

Alport's syndrome

Desc. Progressive renal failure; nerve deafness; ocular abnormalities

Impl. Renal failure in second to third decades; care with renally excreted drugs

Alström syndrome

Desc. Obesity; blindness by 7 yrs of age; hearing loss; diabetes after puberty; glomerulosclerosis

Impl. Renal impairment; management of diabetes and obesity

Amyotonia congenita (infantile muscular atrophy)

Desc. Anterior horn cell degeneration

Impl. Sensitive to thiopental (reduced muscle mass) and respiratory depressants; care with muscle relaxants; at risk for malignant hyperthermia

Amyotrophic lateral sclerosis

Desc. Degeneration of motor neurons

Impl. Avoid succinylcholine; possible K release and cardiac arrest; minimal thiopental and curare; avoid respiratory depressants

Analbuminemia

Desc. Almost absent albumin (4–100 mg/dL)

Impl. Very sensitive to protein-bound drugs

Andersen's disease (glycogen storage disease type IV)

Desc. Debranching enzyme deficiency

Impl. Possibility of hypoglycemia during anesthesia

Anemia of Blackfan and Diamond

Desc. Congenital idiopathic red cell aplasia

Impl. Liver and spleen enlarged; hypersplenism; thrombocytopenia; steroid therapy required

Apert's syndrome (acrocephalosyndactylia)

Desc. Craniosynostosis

Impl. Syndactyly of hands; difficult intubation; possibly raised intracranial pressure; associated congenital heart disease

Arthrogryposis multiplex

Desc. Multiple congenital contractures; stiffness of joints associated with hypoplasia of attached muscles

Impl. Ten percent have congenital heart disease; possible airway problem; at risk for malignant hyperthermia

Asplenia syndrome

Desc. Absent spleen; bilateral visceral right-sidedness

Impl. Very complex cardiovascular anomalies; present with cyanosis and heart failure

Ataxia-telangiectasia

Desc. Cerebellar ataxia; skin and conjunctival telangiectasia; decreased serum IgA and IgE; 10% develop reticuloendothelial malignancy

Impl. Defective immunity—recurrent chest and sinus infections; bronchiectasis; aseptic techniques

Bartter's syndrome[274]

Desc. Hypokalemic hypochloremic metabolic alkalosis, hyperaldosteronism, hyperreninemia, and hyperplasia of the juxtaglomerular apparatus of the kidneys; usually normotensive but may be hypovolemic; may have unstable baroreceptor responses and show marked resistance to vasopressors

Impl. Fluid, acid-base, and electrolyte imbalances along with hemodynamic instability; poses particular problems in anesthetic management

Beckwith's syndrome (infantile gigantism)

Desc. Birth weight >4,000 g; macroglossia and exomphalos; polycythemia visceromegaly in infants

Impl. Older children associated with hepatocellular cancer; persistent severe neonatal hypoglycemia; airway problems

Bowen's syndrome (cerebrohepatorenal syndrome)

Desc. Hypotonia, hepatomegaly, and neonatal jaundice; polycystic kidneys; associated congenital heart disease

Impl. Hypoprothrombinemia; care with renally excreted drugs and muscle relaxants

Carpenter's syndrome

Desc. Obesity; cranial synostosis; associated congenital heart disease; mental retardation; peculiar facies; syndactyly of fingers and toes

Impl. Hypoplastic mandible; possibly difficult intubation

Central core disease

Desc. Muscular dystrophy

Impl. Sensitive to thiopental (reduced muscle mass) and respiratory depressants; care with muscle relaxants; at risk for malignant hyperthermia

Chediak-Higashi syndrome

Desc. Partial albinism immunodeficiency; hepato-splenomegaly

Impl. Steroid therapy; recurrent chest infection; thrombocytopenia—may require platelets

Cherubism

Desc. Tumorous lesion of mandibles and maxillae with intraoral masses; may cause respiratory distress

Impl. Intubation may be extremely difficult; may require tracheostomy for acute respiratory distress; profuse bleeding at surgery

Chotzen's syndrome

Desc. Craniosynostosis

Impl. May be difficult intubation; associated renal anomalies and possible impaired renal excretion of drugs

Christ-Siemens-Touraine syndrome (anhidrotic ectodermal dysplasia)

Desc. Absent sweating, heat intolerance

Impl. Unable to control temperature by sweating; persistent upper respiratory and chest infection due to poor mucus formation

Chronic granulomatous disease

Desc. Inherited disorder of leukocyte function; recurrent infections with nonpathogenic organisms

Impl. Hepatomegaly in 95%; poor pulmonary function; avoid infection—strict asepsis

Collagen disease: dermatomyositis, rheumatoid arthritis, systemic lupus erythematosus, polyarteritis nodosa

Desc. Systemic connective diseases frequently treated with steroids; osteoporosis and fatty infiltration of muscle; variable systemic involvement

Impl. Often have pulmonary infiltration or fibrosis; may have temporomandibular or cricoarytenoid arthritis causing airway and intubation difficulties; anemia common; risk of fat embolism after osteotomy, fracture, or minor trauma; renal involvement common; potential addisonian crises

Colonic atresia

Desc. Congenital atresia of the colon

Impl. Associations: malrotation and other anomalies

Congenital diaphragmatic hernia

Impl. Associations: potentially malrotation, omphalocele, and, occasionally, neural tube defects

Conradi's syndrome

Desc. Chondrodystrophy with contractures, saddle nose, mental retardation; associated congenital heart disease and renal anomalies

Impl. Problems of associated renal and cardiac disease

Cretinism (congenital hypothyroidism)

Desc. Absent thyroid tissue or defective synthesis of thyroxine and goiter

Impl. Airway problems—large tongue, goiter; respiratory center very sensitive to depressants; carbon dioxide retention common; hypoglycemia, hyponatremia, and hypotension; low cardiac output; transfusion poorly tolerated

Cri du chat ("cat's cry") syndrome

Desc. Chromosome 5P abnormal; abnormal, cat-like cry; microcephaly micrognathia; congenital heart disease; hypertelorism exophthalmos

Impl. Airway problems: stridor, laryngomalacia; possibly difficult intubation

Crouzon's disease

Desc. Exophthalmos; hypertelorism; craniosynostosis; hypoplastic mandible

Impl. Possibly difficult intubation; severe blood loss with craniofacial operation

Cutis laxa

Desc. Elastic fiber degeneration, pendulous skin, frequent hernias; emphysema and cor pulmonale; arterial fragility

Impl. Pulmonary infection, emphysema, and cor pulmonale; poor tissues (IV line difficult to maintain); excess of soft tissues around larynx may lead to respiratory obstruction

Cystic fibrosis

Desc. Multisystem involvement

Impl. $\dot{V}/\dot{Q}$ imbalance resulting in hypoxemia; bronchial secretions; recurrent infection; cor pulmonale; liver abnormalities; malabsorption; vitamin K deficiency; coagulopathy

Dermatomyositis

See under Collagen diseases

DiGeorge syndrome (third and fourth arch syndrome)

Desc. Absent thymus and parathyroid glands; immune deficiency; susceptibility to fungal and viral infections; treated by fetal thymic transplants

Impl. Recurrent chest infections; hypoparathyroidism; low calcium and tetany; stridor; aortic arch abnormalities and reduced cardiac output; donor blood irradiated with 3,000 rad to prevent graft-versus-host reaction

Down's syndrome (mongolism)

Desc. Mental retardation; microcephaly; small nasopharynx; hypotonia; congenital heart disease in 60% of patients; duodenal atresia in some; atlantoaxial instability

Impl. Difficult airway (large tongue); risk of airway obstruction; problems of cardiac anomalies; risk of cervical cord injury

Duchenne-type muscular dystrophy

Desc. Muscular dystrophy with frequent cardiac muscle involvement; cardiac failure; usually death in second decade

Impl. As for amyotonia congenita, plus cardiac involvement; minimal drug dosage; avoid respiratory depressants and muscle relaxants, especially succinylcholine; potential postoperative ventilation; at risk for malignant hyperthermia; dantrolene required in the operating room.

Duodenal atresia

Desc. Congenital atresia of the colon

Impl. Possible associations: prematurity, small size for gestational age, trisomy 21, malrotation, tracheoesophageal fistula, annular pancreas, imperforate anus

Edwards' syndrome (trisomy 18 [E])

Desc. Congenital heart disease in 95%; micrognathia in 80%; renal malformations in 50–80%; death usually in infancy

Impl. Possible difficult intubation; care with renally excreted drugs

Ehlers-Danlos syndrome (cutis hyperelastica)

Desc. Collagen abnormality with hyperelasticity and fragile tissues; dissecting aneurysm of aorta; fragility of other blood vessels; bleeding diathesis

Impl. Cardiovascular system; spontaneous rupture of vessels; angiogram (1% mortality); ECG conduction abnormalities; IV line difficult to maintain (hematoma); poor tissues and clotting defect lead to hemorrhage, especially in GI tract; spontaneous pneumothorax

Ellis–van Creveld syndrome (chondroectodermal dysplasia)

Desc. Ectodermal defects, skeletal anomalies; congenital heart disease in 50%

Impl. Chest wall anomalies lead to poor lung function; may have abnormal maxilla and upper lip and hepatosplenomegaly

Epidermolysis bullosa

Desc. Erosions and blisters from minor skin trauma

Impl. Airway (oral lesions, adhesion of tongue); recommended: ketamine or small oral tube to avoid laryngeal trauma; avoid skin trauma from tapes;

history of steroid therapy; possible porphyria (similar skin lesions)

Esophageal atresia and tracheoesophageal fistula

Desc. Congenital atresia of the colon

Impl. Associations: congenital diaphragmatic hernia, congenital heart disease, Vater association, Trisomies 18 and 21

Fabry's disease (diffuse angiokeratoma)

Desc. Lysosomal storage disease; corneal opacities; cardiopulmonary involvement; renal failure

Impl. Hypertension, myocardial ischemia (before third or fourth decade); renal failure (care with renally excreted drugs)

Familial periodic paralysis

Desc. Muscle disease; hypokalemia; attacks of quadriplegia

Impl. Monitor serum K^+; limit use of dextrose; monitor ECG; avoid relaxants

Fanconi's syndrome (renal tubular acidosis)

Desc. Usually secondary to other disease; proximal tubular defect; acidosis K^+ loss; dehydration

Impl. Impaired renal function; treat electrolyte and acid-base abnormalities; look for primary disease (galactosemia, cystinosis, etc.)

Farber's disease (lipogranulomatosis)

Desc. Sphingomyelin deposition; widespread visceral lipogranulomas, especially in the CNS

Impl. Deposits in larynx (careful intubation); generalized systemic involvement leading to cardiac, renal failure

Favism

Desc. G6PD deficiency; hemolytic anemia

Impl. Hemolysis after oxidant drugs (e.g., ASA and sulfa drugs)

Fraser syndrome[222]

Desc. Cardinal features: cryptophthalmus; syndactyly; abnormalities of the nose and ears; syndactyly; atresia or hypoplasia of larynx; high-arched palate; short mentohyoid distance; cardiac anomalies; mental retardation; anomalies of the neuraxis and urinary tract

Impl. Difficult intubation; exclude cardiac defects

Freeman-Sheldon syndrome[329]

Desc. Congenital myopathy and dysplasia; fibrotic contractures of the facial muscles (whistling face); microstomia and micrognathia; ulnar flexion contractures of the hand and equinovarus and valgus deformities of the feet

Impl. Nontriggering agents (?malignant hyperthermia); IV access can be difficult because of limb deformities and thickened subcutaneous tissues; limbs may be encased in casts or splints limiting the available sites for venepuncture; intubation may be difficult

Friedreich's ataxia

Desc. Degeneration of cerebellum and lateral and posterior column of spinal cord; scoliosis; myocardial myopathy and fibrosis

Impl. Heart failure and arrhythmias; care with cardiac depressant drugs

Gastroschisis

Desc. Abdominal wall defect through which abdominal viscera protrude; no membranous covering

Impl. Patient may be small for gestational age; may have bowel atresias

Gaucher's disease

Desc. Cerebroside accumulation in CNS, liver, spleen, and so forth.

Impl. Pulmonary disease from aspiration (pseudobulbar palsy); hepatosplenomegaly, hypersplenism; possible platelet deficiency

Glanzmann's disease (thrombasthenia)

Desc. Platelet adenosine diphosphate; reduced-abnormal function

Impl. No specific therapy for bleeding; platelet transfusion disappointing; history of steroids

Goldenhar's syndrome (oculoauriculovertebral dysplasia)

Desc. Unilateral facial hypoplasia; congenital heart disease in 20%; mandibular hypoplasia in 60%

Impl. Difficult airway and intubation; problems of associated cardiac disease

Gorlin-Goltz syndrome (focal dermal hypoplasia)

Desc. Hernias, prolapse, and so forth; congenital heart disease; renal anomalies

Impl. Asymmetry of head (difficult airway)

Grönblad-Strandberg syndrome (pseudoxanthoma elasticum)

Desc. Degeneration of elastic tissue in skin, eye, and cardiovascular system

Impl. Rupture of arteries, especially in gastrointestinal tract; hypertension; arterial calcification; occlusion of cerebral and coronary arteries; difficult maintenance of IV cannula

Guillain-Barré syndrome (acute idiopathic polyneuritis)

Desc. Acute polyneuropathy; progressive peripheral neuritis often involving cranial nerves; bulbar palsy with hypoventilation and hypotension

Impl. Avoid succinylcholine for K^+ release; may require tracheostomy, mechanical ventilation, and support of blood pressure

Hand-Schüller-Christian disease (histiocytosis X)

Desc. Histiocytic granulomas in bones and viscera (larynx, lungs, liver, and spleen)

Impl. Laryngeal fibrosis; pulmonary failure (diffuse or hilar infiltration); respiratory failure and cor pulmonale; hypersplenism and pancytopenia; liver involvement; diabetes insipidus if sella turcica involved; history of steroids; benign intracranial hypertension; tooth loss

Hermansky-Pudlak syndrome

Desc. Albinism, bleeding diathesis

Impl. Platelet abnormality; try platelet transfusion; no specific treatment

Holt-Oram syndrome (heart-hand syndrome)

Desc. Upper limb abnormalities; congenital heart disease (atrioseptal defect); possibly sudden death from pulmonary embolus or coronary occlusion

Impl. Problems of cardiac defect

Homocystinuria

Desc. Inborn error of metabolism; thromboembolic phenomena due to intimal thickening; ectopia lentis, osteoporosis, and kyphoscoliosis

Impl. Dextran 70 to reduce viscosity and platelet adhesiveness; increase peripheral perfusion; angiography may precipitate thrombosis, including coronary thrombosis

Hunter's syndrome (mucopolysaccharidosis II)

Desc. Stiff joints, dwarfing, hepatosplenomegaly; pectus excavatum, and kyphoscoliosis; valvular and coronary heart disease

Impl. Upper airway obstruction due to infiltration of lymphoid tissue and larynx; pneumonias; possible hypersplenism; cardiac failure

Hurler's syndrome (mucopolysaccharidosis I)

Desc. Pulmonary hypertension; death usually before age 10 yrs from respiratory and cardiac failure

Impl. As for Hunter's syndrome, but more severe; frequent upper respiratory infection; abnormal tracheobronchial cartilages; severe coronary artery disease at early age; valvular and myocardial involvement

Ileal atresia

Impl. May be premature and may have an imperforate anus

Imperforate anus

Impl. Vater association, Meckel's diverticulum, and trisomy 21 may be associated with imperforate anus

Jejunal atresia

Impl. May be premature and have associated malrotation and biliary atresia

Jervell and Lange-Nielsen syndrome (cardioauditory syndrome)

Desc. Cardiac conduction defects; deafness

Impl. Syncope, arrhythmias; large T waves and prolonged QT interval on ECG; may need digoxin or propranolol (or both) or pacemaker

Jeune's syndrome (asphyxiating thoracic dystrophy)

Desc. Narrow, immobile thorax; respiratory failure; nephritis

Impl. Severe restrictive lung disease; may require postoperative ventilatory support

Kartagener's syndrome (immotile cilia syndrome)
Desc. Situs inversus, immotile cilia, deficient mucociliary clearance, sinusitis, otitis media, chronic bronchitis
Impl. Chronic respiratory and sinus infection

Kasabach-Merritt syndrome
Desc. Hemangioma and thrombocytopenia; average age at death: 5 wks
Impl. Hemangioma suddenly increases in size with associated severe thrombocytopenia and hemorrhage; replace blood loss, transfuse platelets; splenectomy; steroids

Klippel-Feil syndrome
Desc. Congenital fusion of two or more cervical vertebrae, leading to neck rigidity
Impl. Difficult airway and intubation

Klippel-Trenaunay syndrome (angio-osteohypertrophy)
Desc. Usually unilateral; arteriovenous fistulas, thrombocytopenia
Impl. Arteriovenous fistulas and anemia to high cardiac output state; thrombocytopenia in visceral hemangiomas

Larsen's syndrome
Desc. Multiple congenital dislocations; connective tissue defect; poor cartilage in rib cage, epiglottis, arytenoids
Impl. Possible difficult intubation; chronic respiratory problems

Laurence-Moon-Biedl syndrome

Desc. Obesity, retinitis pigmentosa; polydactyly; mental retardation

Impl. May be associated with cardiac defects, renal disease, and occasionally diabetes insipidus

Leopard syndrome

Desc. Multiple large freckles; congenital heart disease; ECG anomalies (aberrant conduction); hypertelorism

Impl. 95% pulmonary stenosis

Leprechaunism

Desc. Failure to thrive; endocrine disorders; severe mental retardation

Impl. Hypoglycemia due to hyperinsulinism from hyperplastic islet of Langerhans; renal tubular defects (impaired renal function)

Lesch-Nyhan syndrome

Desc. Hyperuricemia and mental retardation; renal failure by age 10 yrs

Impl. High serum uric acid leads to red cell damage and renal stones; care with renally excreted drugs

Letterer-Siwe disease (histiocytosis X)

Desc. Histiocytic granulomas in viscera and bones; clinical course similar to acute leukemia

Impl. Pancytopenia-anemia and purpura hemorrhage; pulmonary infiltration; hepatic involvement; gingival inflammation and necrosis; loss of teeth

Lipodystrophy (total lipoatrophy)

Desc. Generalized loss of all body fat; fatty, fibrotic liver, portal hypertension and splenomegaly; nephropathy; diabetes

Impl. Liver failure (avoid halothane and drugs metabolized by liver); hypersplenism (anemia and thrombocytopenia); possible renal failure; usual diabetic precautions

Lowe syndrome (oculocerebrorenal syndrome)

Desc. Men only; cataract and glaucoma; mental retardation; hypotonia; renal acidosis, proteinuria, osteoporosis, and rickets

Impl. Check electrolyte and acid-base balance; check serum Ca^{++} (treated with vitamin D and Ca^{++}); care with renally excreted drugs

Lyme disease

Impl. Arrhythmias, myocarditis

Maffucci's syndrome

Desc. Enchondromatosis and hemangiomas with malignant change

Impl. Pathologic fractures; gastrointestinal bleeding from hemangiomas; orthostatic hypotension; may be sensitive to vasodilator drugs

Maple syrup urine disease (branched-chain ketonuria)

Desc. Amino acid disturbance treated by diet only; severe neurologic damage and respiratory disturbances

Impl. General supportive measures

Marfan syndrome (arachnodactyly)

Desc. Connective tissue disorder; dilatation of aortic root leads to aortic insufficiency; aortic, thoracic, or abdominal aneurysm; pulmonary artery, mitral valve involved; kyphoscoliosis, pectus excavatum, lung cysts; joint instability and dislocation

Impl. Care with myocardial depressant drugs; beware of possible dissection of aorta; lung function poor; possible pneumothorax; care in positioning (easily dislocated joints)

Maroteaux-Lamy syndrome (mucopolysaccharidosis IV)

Desc. Myocardial involvement; kyphoscoliosis and chest infection; hepatosplenomegaly

Impl. Heart failure by age 20 yrs; care with cardiac depressant drugs; chronic respiratory infection with poor lung reserve; hypersplenism, anemia, thrombocytopenia

McArdle's disease

Desc. Glycogen storage disease type V

Impl. Muscles affected, including cardiac muscle; care with cardiac depressant drugs

Meckel's syndrome

Desc. Microcephaly, micrognathia, and cleft epiglottis; congenital heart disease; renal dysplasia

Impl. Intubation may be difficult; cardiac problems; renal failure in infancy—care with renally excreted drugs

Meconium ileus

Desc. Bowel obstruction by thick stringy mucus at the level of the ileum

Impl. May have associated cystic fibrosis

Median cleft face syndrome

Desc. Varying degrees of cleft face; frontal lipomas and dermoids

Impl. Possible intubation difficulties caused by cleft nose, lip, and palate

Melas syndrome[368]

Desc. Mitochondrial dysfunction (lactic acid, ragged-red fibers), seizures, dementia, headaches, stroke-like episodes, nephropathy, peripheral neuropathy

Impl. Myopathy (sensitivity to neuromuscular blockers, ?hyperkalemia after succinylcholine, ?malignant hyperthermia); acidosis; check for conduction defects and cardiomyopathies

Möbius' syndrome (congenital facial diplegia)

Desc. Associated limb deformities, micrognathia; agenesis of cranial motor nuclei

Impl. Feeding difficulties and aspiration may cause chronic pulmonary problems; may be difficult to intubate

Morquio-Ullrich syndrome (mucopolysaccharidosis IV)

Desc. Severe dwarfing; aortic incompetence; thoracic deformities; unstable atlantoaxial joint

Impl. Cardiorespiratory symptoms by second decade; severe kyphoscoliosis with poor lung function; all develop spinal cord damage from atlanto-occipital subluxation

Moschcowitz's disease (thrombotic thrombocytopenic purpura)

Desc. Hemolytic anemia and thrombocytopenia; small vessel disease; neurologic damage and renal disease; treatment: splenectomy and steroids

Impl. History of steroid therapy; care with renally excreted drugs if kidneys affected

Multiple pterygium syndrome[330]

Desc. Micrognathia, ankyloglossia, cleft palate, and pterygium colli (bands across the neck causing flexion and rotation); neck extension significantly limited; airway deformities (posterior pharynx may not be visualized); muscular ventricular septal defect, camptodactyly, clubfoot deformities, and pterygia across the elbows, axilla, and popliteal fossae

Impl. Very difficult airway problems

Myasthenia congenita

Desc. Like adult myasthenia gravis

Impl. Avoid respiratory depressants and muscle relaxants; may require postoperative ventilation;

problems of anticholinesterase therapy pre- and postoperatively; possibility of cholinergic crisis

Myositis ossificans (fibrodysplasia ossificans)

Desc. Bony infiltration of tendons, fascia, aponeuroses, and muscle

Impl. Airway and intubation problems if neck rigid; thoracic involvement leads to aspiration and asphyxia, lung pathology, and grossly reduced thoracic compliance

Myotonia congenita (Thomsen's disease)

Desc. Decreased ability to relax muscles after contraction; diffuse hypertrophy of muscle

Impl. Avoid relaxants and depressants as for myotonic dystrophy, although this is a more benign disease; nonprogressive; at risk for malignant hyperthermia

Myotonic dystrophy (myotonia dystrophica)

Desc. Weakness and myotonia; ptosis, cataracts, partial baldness, and gonadal atrophy; cardiac conduction defects and arrhythmias; impaired ventilation

Impl. Avoid succinylcholine (causes myotonia in 50%); nondepolarizing drugs ineffective for relaxing myotonia; neostigmine induces myotonia; monitor ECG; extremely sensitive to respiratory depressants (use regional or inhalation agents); halothane may cause postoperative shivering and myotonia; pulmonary complications due to poor cough; at risk for malignant hyperthermia

Niemann-Pick disease

Desc. Sphingomyelin and cholesterol accumulation in CNS, marrow, liver, and spleen; diffuse infiltration of lungs; epilepsy, ataxia, and mental retardation

Impl. Anemia and thrombocytopenia due to marrow and spleen involvement; pulmonary insufficiency pneumonia

Noack's syndrome

Desc. Craniosynostosis and digital anomalies; obesity

Impl. May be difficult to intubate because of skull deformity

Noonan's syndrome (formerly called *male Turner's syndrome*)

Desc. Short stature, mental retardation, congenital heart disease, and micrognathia; hydronephrosis or hypoplasia of kidneys

Impl. Usually pulmonary stenosis or patent ductus arteriosus and tetralogy; care with renally excreted drugs if kidneys affected

Ollier's disease (enchondromatosis)

Desc. Multiple chondromas within bones, usually unilateral; pathologic fractures

Impl. With cavernous hemangioma: described as Maffucci's syndrome; care with positioning

Omphalocele

Impl. 30% have associated anomalies such as Beckwith-Wiedemann syndrome; imperforate anus;

meningocele; congenital heart disease; ileal atresia; bladder extrophy; trisomies 13, 18, or 21; pulmonary hypoplasia; spinal skeletal defects.

Orofaciodigital syndrome

Desc. Cleft lip and palate, lobed tongue; hypoplastic mandible and maxilla; digital anomalies; hydrocephalus, polycystic kidneys

Impl. Difficult airway and intubation; possible renal failure

Oro-palato-facial syndrome[241]

Desc. Small mouth, cleft palate, anomalies of cervical spine

Impl. Difficult airway and intubation

Osler-Weber-Rendu disease (hemorrhagic telangiectasia)

Desc. No coagulation abnormalities; associated pulmonary arteriovenous fistula

Impl. Blood loss may be impossible to control; IV line may be difficult to maintain due to poor tissues; recurrent chest infection; dyspnea, cyanosis, and clubbing possible

Osteogenesis imperfecta (fragilitas ossium)

Desc. I. Congenita (stillborn or rapidly fatal)
II. Tarda (pathologic fractures); osteoporosis leads to kyphoscoliosis

Impl. Lung pathology due to chest deformity; subcutaneous hemorrhage due to fragile vessels; carious and easily broken teeth due to dentin deficiency;

extreme care in positioning; at risk for malignant hyperthermia

Oto-palato-digital syndrome[240]

Desc. Frontal bossing, hypertelorism, midfacial hypoplasia, micrognathism, shortening of the distal phalanges on both hands and feet

Impl. Significant airway problems

Paramyotonia congenita (Eulenburg's disease)

Desc. Myotonia on exposure to cold; paroxysmal weakness; serum K^+ may be high or low

Impl. Anesthesia as for myotonic dystrophy; also care with K^+ level; at risk for malignant hyperthermia

Patau's syndrome (trisomy 13)

Desc. Mental retardation; microcephaly, micrognathia, or dextrocardia (or all three); cleft lip or cleft palate; congenital heart disease; usually fatal by age 3 yrs

Impl. Difficult intubation; usually ventricular septal defect

Pendred's syndrome

Desc. Deafness and goiter; incomplete block of thyroxine production

Impl. May be euthyroid or hypothyroid; similar to cretinism

Pierre Robin syndrome

Desc. Cleft palate, micrognathia, glossoptosis; associated congenital heart disease may occur

Impl. Newborn may asphyxiate; may require tongue suture, intubation, or tracheostomy; may be very difficult to intubate; awake intubation

Polyarteritis nodosa

See under Collagen diseases

Polycystic kidneys

Desc. Associated cysts in liver, pancreas, spleen, lungs, bladder, thyroid in 33%; cerebral aneurysm in 15%

Impl. Care with renally excreted drugs; lung cysts; may lead to pneumothorax; avoid hypertension because of possible cerebral aneurysm

Polycystic liver

Desc. Familial: 60% have polycystic kidneys, lungs, and pancreas

Impl. Usually liver function not impaired until late (fibrosis, splenomegaly, esophageal varices, etc.); renal failure and lung cysts possible

Polysplenia

Desc. Bilateral visceral left-sidedness

Impl. Complex cardiac anomalies common; atrioseptal defect and endocardial cushion defects; usually not so complex as in asplenia

Pompe's disease (glycogen storage II)

Desc. Muscle deposits—severe hypotonicity; short PR interval, arrhythmias, massive cardiomegaly; cardiac failure; death before age 2 yrs

Impl. Extreme care; avoid respiratory depressants, muscle relaxants, cardiac depressants; possible airway problem due to large tongue

Porphyria

Desc. Paralysis, psychiatric disorder; autonomic imbalance (hypertension and tachycardia); abdominal pain precipitated by drugs, infections, and so forth

Impl. Avoid: barbiturates (including thiopental), sedatives (meprobamate, Librium, glutethimide, carbromal), hydroxydione (steroid anesthetic), nikethamide, hydantoin derivatives, sulfonamides, antipyretics, hypoglycemic agents; no harmful effects expected with opiates, phenothiazines, local anesthetics, N_2O, halothane, isoflurane, muscle relaxants, atropine, neostigmine, pentolinium, and corticosteroids

Prader-Willi syndrome

Desc. Neonate: hypotonia, poor feeding, absent reflexes; second phase: hyperactive, uncontrollable polyphagia, mental retardation

Impl. Obesity of extreme proportions leading to cardiopulmonary failure

Progeria (Hutchinson-Gilford syndrome)

Desc. Premature aging starts between ages 6 mos to 3 yrs; cardiac disease (ischemia, hypertension, and cardiomegaly)

Impl. Anesthesia as for adults with myocardial ischemia

Prune-belly syndrome

Desc. Agenesis of abdominal musculature, renal anomalies, cryptorchidism

Impl. Poor cough (respiratory infections); respiration requires accessory muscles; treat as full stomach; intubate and assist or control ventilation; progressive failure and urinary tract infection frequent

Rheumatoid arthritis

Desc. In addition to skeletal involvement, may have pericarditis
See also under Collagen diseases

Rieger's syndrome

Desc. Myotonic dystrophy and other myopathies; hypoplasia of maxilla, abnormal teeth; mental retardation; occasional imperforate anus

Impl. Anesthetic requirements dictated by associated muscle disease (see amyotonia congenita, myotonic dystrophy); at risk for malignant hyperthermia

Riley-Day syndrome (familial dysautonomia)

Desc. Deficiency of dopamine hydroxylase; hyper and hypotensive attacks, absent lacrimation, abnormal sweating; insensitive to pain; poor suckling and swallowing

Impl. Emotional lability; recurrent aspiration, pneumonia, and chronic lung disease; labile blood pressure; sensitive to adrenergic and cholinergic drugs; respiratory center insensitive to CO_2; avoid respiratory depressants

Rubenstein-Taybi syndrome[221]

Desc. Mental retardation; broad thumbs and third toes; craniofacial abnormalities; recurrent respiratory infections and congenital heart disease (30%)

Impl. Minor difficulties with intubation; easy desaturation

Russel-Silver syndrome[305]

Desc. A form of dwarfism characterized by intrauterine growth retardation and subsequent severe postnatal growth impairment, dysmorphic facial features (including mandibular and facial hypoplasia), limb asymmetry, and a constellation of endocrine abnormalities including hypoglycemia and various patterns of hypogonadism

Impl. Management concerns: mask ventilation, tracheal intubation, temperature regulation, dosing of relaxants, emergence from anesthesia, and glucose homeostasis; possible concomitant associations: heart disease, hypopituitarism, and adrenal insufficiency

Sanfilippo's syndrome (mucopolysaccharidosis III)

Desc. CNS malfunction in childhood progresses to mental retardation and dementia; no hepatosplenomegaly or cardiac problems

Impl. No anesthetic problems described; emotional disturbance, agitation, and dementia

Schwartz-Jampel syndrome[220]

Desc. Clinical features: appear soon after birth and progress to mid-adolescence (when they become static); microstomia and limited joint motility from increased muscle tone, which causes rigidity; mask-like facies, blepharophimosis, and pursed mouth; short stature, kyphoscoliosis, lumbar lordosis, bowed long bones, pes planus, and ankle valgus

Impl. Difficulties with intubation: microstomia and rigidity (none reported so far, however); thermoregulatory dysfunction; possible limited chest-wall expansion because of rigidity caused by compromised lung function; at risk for malignant hyperthermia

Scleroderma

Desc. Diffuse cutaneous stiffening; plastic surgery required for contractures and constrictions

Impl. Scarring of face and mouth (difficult airway and intubation); chest restriction (poor compliance); diffuse pulmonary fibrosis; hypoxia; veins often invisible and impalpable; cardiac fibrosis or cor pulmonale; history of steroid therapy

Sebaceous nevi (linear)

Desc. Linear nevi from forehead to nose; hydrocephalus, mental retardation; associated with coarctation and hypoplasia of aorta

Impl. Cardiovascular complications

Shy-Drager syndrome

Desc. Orthostatic hypotension; diffuse degeneration of CNS and autonomic nervous system; decreased sweating; hypersensitive to angiotensin and epinephrine

Impl. Labile pulse and blood pressure possibly due to defective baroreceptor response; treat hypotension with infusion; phenylephrine hydrochloride (Neo-Synephrine)

Silver's syndrome

Desc. Short stature, skeletal asymmetry; micrognathia; abnormal sexual development

Impl. Intubation possibly difficult

Sipple's syndrome (multiple endocrine adenomatosis type II)

Desc. Pheochromocytoma and medullary thyroid carcinoma; parathyroid adenoma; CNS tumors; schwannoma of mediastinum associated; Cushing's disease

Impl. Management of pheochromocytoma (75% bilateral); problems of multiple endocrine disorders

Smith-Lemli-Opitz syndrome

Desc. Mental retardation; genital and skeletal anomalies (micrognathia); thymic hypoplasia

Impl. Airway and intubation problems; pneumonia, possible increased susceptibility to infection

Sotos' syndrome (cerebral gigantism)

Desc. Acromegalic features; dilated ventricles but normal intracranial pressure

Impl. All features nonprogressive; possible airway problems due to acromegalic skull; no other described problems

Stevens-Johnson syndrome

Desc. Erythema multiforme, urticarial lesions, and erosions of mouth, eyes, genitalia; possible hypersensitivity to exogenous agents (e.g., drugs, infections)

Impl. Oral lesions—avoid intubation, esophageal stethoscope; monitoring difficult because of skin lesions; fibrillation, myocarditis, pericarditis occur; febrile episodes; pleural blebs and pneumothorax may occur

Sturge-Weber syndrome

Desc. Cavernous angioma over third division of fifth cranial nerve; intracranial calcification, convulsions, and possible progressive neurologic deficit

Impl. No specific anesthetic problems

Supravalvular aortic stenosis syndrome (idiopathic infantile hypercalcemia; Williams syndrome)

Desc. Hypercalcemia and mental retardation; abnormal facies; dyspnea and angina; therapy: low-calcium diet, steroids; cardiac surgery

Impl. Fixed cardiac output and ischemia; history of steroids; monitor serum Ca^{++}

Systemic lupus erythematosus

See under Collagen diseases

Tangier disease (analphalipoproteinemia)

Desc. Low serum cholesterol; orange tonsils and rectal mucosa; splenomegaly; 50% neurologic abnormality; premature coronary disease

Impl. Anemia and thrombocytopenia due to hypersplenism; abnormal EMG (care with muscle relaxants); premature ischemic heart disease

Tay-Sachs disease

Desc. Gangliosidosis; blindness and progressive dementia; degeneration of CNS

Impl. No described anesthetic hazard; progressive neurologic loss leads to respiratory complications; treatment: supportive measures

Thrombocytopenia with absent radius

Desc. Episodic thrombocytopenia precipitated by stress, infection, surgery, and so forth; low platelets improve to normal by adulthood; congenital heart disease in 30%

Impl. Platelet transfusion for surgery or bleeding (35–40% die in first year of intracranial hemorrhage); avoid elective surgery in first year

Treacher Collins syndrome (mandibulofacial dysostosis)

Desc. Micrognathia and aplastic zygomatic arches; microstomia, choanal atresia; congenital heart disease may occur

Impl. Possible airway and intubation difficulties; less severe than Pierre Robin deformity

Tuberous sclerosis

Desc. Adenoma sebaceum of skin, epilepsy, and mental retardation; intracranial calcification in 50%; hamartomas in lungs, kidneys, and heart

Impl. Kidneys: pyelonephritis and renal failure; care with renally excreted drugs; lungs: possible rupture of lung cysts; possible cardiac arrhythmia

Turner's syndrome

Desc. XO chromosome; micrognathia, coarctation, dissecting aneurysm of aorta, or pulmonary stenosis; renal anomalies in more than 50%

Impl. Possibly difficult intubation; cardiovascular abnormality; possible renal disease: care with renally excreted drugs

Urbach-Wiethe disease (cutaneomucosal hyalinosis)

Desc. Type of histiocytosis (see Hand-Schüller-Christian disease); hoarseness or aphonia; hyaline deposits in larynx and pharynx

Impl. Cautious intubation

von Gierke's disease

Desc. Glycogen storage disease type I; hepatomegaly, enlarged kidneys, severe attacks of hypoglycemia

Impl. Monitor blood sugar and acid-base balance (IV glucose infusion); diazoxide for hypoglycemia

von Hippel–Lindau disease

Desc. Retinal or CNS hemangioblastoma (posterior fossa or spinal cord); associated with pheochromocytoma, renal, pancreatic, or hepatic cysts

Impl. Problems associated with pheochromocytoma and renal and hepatic pathology

von Recklinghausen's disease (neurofibromatosis)

Desc. Café au lait spots; tumors in all parts of CNS; peripheral tumors associated with nerve trunks; increased incidence of pheochromocytoma; 50% kyphoscoliosis; honeycomb cystic lung changes; renal artery dysplasia and hypertension

Impl. Screen for pheochromocytoma (urinary vanillylmandelic acid); should be investigated for lung function; tumors may occur in larynx and right ventricle outflow tract; care with renally excreted drugs if kidneys involved

von Willebrand's disease (pseudohemophilia)

Desc. Prolonged bleeding time (decreased factor VIII activity) due to defective platelet adhesiveness; ?capillary abnormality

Impl. Bleeding can be controlled by fresh or fresh frozen plasma, cryoprecipitate; avoid salicylate therapy (effect on platelets; possible gastrointestinal bleeding)

Weber-Christian disease (chronic nonsuppurative panniculitis)

Desc. Necrosis of fat in any location, including retroperitoneal, pericardial, and meningeal

Impl. Involvement of retroperitoneal tissues may cause acute or chronic adrenal insufficiency (of pericardium leads to restrictive pericarditis, of meninges causes convulsions); avoid trauma to fat by heat, cold, or pressure

Welander muscular atrophy

Desc. Initial involvement of peripheral muscles; prognosis good for life, poor for ambulation; cardiac arrhythmias and congestive heart failure may occur

Impl. May require spinal fusion; extreme care with thiopental, muscle relaxants; avoid respiratory depressant drugs

Werdnig-Hoffmann disease

Desc. Infantile muscular atrophy more severe than Welander muscular atrophy; feeding difficulties, aspiration, usually death before puberty

Impl. Chronic respiratory problems; minimal anesthesia required; avoid muscle relaxants and respiratory depressant drugs; ventilatory support may be required; weaning may be difficult

Wermer's syndrome (multiple endocrine adenomatosis type I)

Desc. Hyperparathyroidism; tumors of pituitary and pancreatic islet cells; gastric ulcer; occasionally have carcinoid tumors of bronchial tree

Impl. Renal failure due to stones; hypoglycemia from hyperinsulinism

Werner's syndrome

Desc. Premature aging, diabetes; early cataracts; mental retardation in 50%; bony lesions like osteomyelitis; cardiac infarction and failure

Impl. Anesthesia as for adult with myocardial ischemia

Wilson's disease (hepatolenticular degeneration)

Desc. Decreased ceruloplasmin causes abnormal copper deposits especially in liver and CNS motor nuclei; renal tubular acidosis

Impl. Hepatic failure due to fibrosis

Wiskott-Aldrich syndrome

Desc. Immunodeficiency with thrombocytopenia; 100% have low platelets, absent isohemagglutinins; high IgA and low IgM; eczema; asthma

Impl. Blood transfusion and platelets may be required; bone marrow transplantation has been used; all blood products must be irradiated with 3,000 rad to prevent graft-versus-host reaction; avoid contamination; death often from generalized herpes or infection by nonpathogenic organisms

Wolff-Parkinson-White syndrome

Desc. ECG abnormalities: short PR interval, prolonged QRS with phasic variation in 40% of patients; associated with many cardiac defects; anomalous conduction path between atria and ventricles

Impl. Scopolamine preferred to atropine as drying agent; tachycardia due to atropine or apprehension may change ECG with ST segment depression; paroxysmal supraventricular tachycardia on induction of anesthesia or during cardiac surgery has been reported; should be treated with digitalis, propranolol, and pacemaker, if necessary; neostigmine may accentuate the Wolff-Parkinson-White pattern

Wolman disease (familial xanthomatosis)

Desc. Adrenal calcification; resembles Niemann-Pick disease with hepatosplenomegaly and hypersplenism; involvement of other tissues from foam cells, including myocardium

Impl. Anemia and thrombocytopenia; platelet transfusion successful only postsplenectomy

NOTES

NOTES

NOTES

References

1. Rice LJ. Pain Management in Children. In MA Ashburn, PG Fine, TH Stanley (eds), Pain Management in Anesthesiology. Boston: Kluwer, 1998;153–166.
2. DeBock T, Davis P, Tome J, et al. Effect of premedication and arterial oxygen saturation in children with congenital heart disease. J Cardiothoracic Anesth 1990;4:425–429.
3. Report of the Committee on Infectious Diseases of the American Academy of Pediatrics (20th ed). Elk Grove Village, IL: American Academy of Pediatrics, 1986.
4. Chameides L, Hazinski MF (eds). American Heart Association. Pediatric Advanced Life Support. Dallas: Subcommittee on Pediatric Resuscitation, 1997;6.1–6.17.
5. American Heart Association. Standards and guidelines for cardiopulmonary resuscitation (CPR) and emergency cardiac care (ECC). JAMA 1986;255:2905.
6. Rose DK, Frose AB. The regulation of $Paco_2$ during controlled ventilation in children with a T-piece. Can J Anaesth 1979;26:104.
7. Bain JA, Spoerel WE. Flow requirements for a modified Mapleson D system during controlled ventilation. Can J Anaesth 1973;20:629.
8. Goetting MG, Paradis NA. High dose epinephrine improves outcome from pediatric cardiac arrest. Ann Emerg Med 1991;20:22–26.
9. Graves S. Electrolyte and Fluid Therapy in Children. Annual American Society of Anesthesiologists Refresher Courses. Park Ridge, IL: American Society of Anesthesiologists, 1981. Lecture #114.
10. Moore RA. Perioperative Care of the Child with Congenital Cardiac Disease. In CL Lake (ed), Pediatric Cardiac Anesthesia. East Norwalk, CT: Appleton & Lange, 1993;217.

11. Wiley IF, Kopkei JA. A revised rule-of-thumb for predicting the hematocrit rise in premature infants following packed red blood cell transfusion. Clin Lab Haematol 1986;8:93.
12. Viby-Mogensen J, Howardly-Hansen P, Chraemmer-Jorgensen B, et al. Post-tetanic count (PTC): a new method of evaluating an intense nondepolarizing neuromuscular blockade. Anesthesiology 1981;55:458.
13. Viby-Mogensen J. Clinical assessment of neuromuscular transmission. Br J Anaesth 1982;54:209.
14. Muchhal KK, Viby-Mogensen J, Fernando PU, et al. Evaluation of intense neuromuscular blockade caused by vecuronium using post-tetanic count (PTC). Anesthesiology 1987;66:846.
15. Bonsu AK, Viby-Mogensen J, Fernando PU, et al. Relationship of post-tetanic count and train-of-four response during intense neuromuscular blockade caused by atracurium. Br J Anaesth 1987;59:1089.
16. Brandom BW, Bikhazi G, Ginsberg B, Kenaan CA. Org-9487 in neonates, infants and toddlers anesthetized with nitrous oxide-halothane. In: Program and abstracts of the 1998 annual meeting of the Society for Pediatric Anesthesia; February 19, 1998; Pheonix, AZ. Abstract 60.
17. Markakis DA, Sayson SC, Schreiner MS. Insertion of the laryngeal mask airway in awake infants with the Robin sequence. Anesth Analg 1992;79:822.
18. Varner PD, Ebert JP, McKay RD, et al. Methohexital sedation of children undergoing CT scan. Anesth Analg 1985;64:643.
19. Hinkle AJ. Percutaneous inguinal block for the outpatient management of post-herniorrhaphy pain in children. Anesthesiology 1987;67:411.
20. Carrel ED, Eyring EJ. Intravenous regional anesthesia for childhood fractures. J Trauma 1971;11:301.
21. Armitage EN. Pediatric Regional Anaesthesia. In JAW Wildsmith, EN Armitage (eds), Principles and Practice of Regional Anesthesia. London: Churchill Livingstone, 1993;223–232.
22. Berde CB. Convulsions associated with pediatric regional anesthesia. Anesth Analg 1992;75:164.
23. Bromage PR. Ageing and epidural dose requirements: segmental spread and predictability of epidural analgesia in youth and extreme age. Br J Anaesth 1969;41:1016.

24. Melman E, Penuelas JA, Marrufo J. Regional anesthesia in children. Anesth Analg 1975;54:387.
25. Dalens B, Tanguy A, Haberer J. Lumbar epidural anesthesia for operative and postoperative pain relief in infants an young children. Anesth Analg 1986;65:1069–1073.
26. Gregory GA. Monitoring During Surgery. In GA Gregory (ed), Pediatric Anesthesia. New York: Churchill Livingstone, 1983;391.
27. Beasley JM, Jones EF. Anatomical and Physiological Considerations. In JM Beasley, EF Jones (eds), A Guide to Paediatric Anaesthesia. Oxford, UK: Blackwell, 1980;11.
28. Lerman J, Robinson S, Willis MM, Gregory GA. Anesthetic requirements for halothane in young children 0–1 months and 1–6 months of age. Anesthesiology 1983;59:421.
29. Cameron CB, Robinson S, Gregory GA. The MAC of isoflurane in children. Anesth Analg 1984;63:418.
30. de Jongh RH, Eger EI. MAC expanded: AD50 and AD95 values of common inhalation anesthetics in man. Anesthesiology 1975; 42:384.
31. American Heart Association. Pediatric advanced life support. JAMA 1992;268:2262.
32. Weldon BC, Watcha MF, White PF. Oral midazolam in children: effect of time and adjunctive therapy. Anesth Analg 1992;75:51.
33. Bell C, Kain ZN, Hughes C. Appendix A. In C Bell, ZN Kain, C Hughes (eds), The Pediatric Anesthesia Handbook. St. Louis: Mosby–Year Book, 1997;620.
34. McMillan CO, Spahr-Schopfer IA, Sickish N, et al. Premedication of children with oral midazolam. Can J Anaesth 1993;40:726–729.
35. Taketomo CK, Hodding JH, Kraus DM. Pediatric Dosage Handbook. Hudson, OH: Lexi-Corp, 1996;706.
36. Chameides L, Hazinski MF (eds). Pediatric Advanced Life Support. Subcommittee on Pediatric Resuscitation. Cardiac Rhythm Disturbances. Dallas: American Heart Association. 1997;7.1–7.16.
37. Saarnivaara L, Lindgren L, Klemola UM. Comparison of chloral hydrate and midazolam by mouth as premedicants in children undergoing otolaryngeal surgery. Br J Anaesth 1988;61:390.
38. Brzustowicz RM, Nelson DA, Betts EK, et al. Efficacy of oral premedication in pediatric outpatient surgery. Anesthesiology 1984;60:475.

39. Lerman J, Eustis S, Smith DR. Effect of droperidol pretreatment on postanesthetic vomiting in children undergoing strabismus surgery. Anesthesiology 1986;65:322.
40. Christensen S, Farrow-Gillespie A, Lerman J. Incidence of emesis and postanesthetic recovery after strabismus surgery in children: a comparison of droperidol and lidocaine. Anesthesiology 1989; 70:251.
41. Hendrickson M, Myre L, Johnson DG, et al. Postoperative analgesia in children: a prospective study of intermittent intramuscular injection versus continuous intravenous infusion of morphine. J Pediatr Surg 1990;25:185.
42. Jones SE, Beasley JM, Macfarlane DW, et al. Intrathecal morphine for postoperative pain relief in children. Br J Anaesth 1984;6:137.
43. Rosen KR, Rosen DA. Caudal morphine for control of pain following open heart surgery in children. Anesthesiology 1989;70:418.
44. Attia J, Ecoffey C, Sandouk P, et al. Epidural morphine in children: pharmacokinetics and CO_2 sensitivity. Anesthesiology 1986;65:590.
45. Audanaert SM, Vickers H, Burgess RC. Axillary block for vascular insufficiency after repair of radial club hands in an infant. Anesthesiology 1991;74:368.
46. Gordon JB, Yeager M. Management of the Child with Malignant Disease in the Pediatric Intensive Care Unit. In MC Rogers (ed), Textbook of Pediatric Intensive Care. Baltimore: Williams & Wilkins, 1992;1403–1440.
47. Lawless S, Burckhart G, Diven W, et al. Amrinone pharmacokinetics in neonates and infants. J Clin Pharmacol 1988;28:283.
48. Lockhart CH, Nelson WL. The relationship of ketamine requirements to age in pediatric patients. Anesthesiology 1974;40:507.
49. Taylor G, Boswell MV. Continuous epidural infusion of low dose morphine for postoperative analgesia in children. Anesthesiology 1991;75A:A937.
50. Sarner JB, Brandom BW, Dong ML, et al. Clinical pharmacology of pipecuronium in infants and children during halothane anesthesia. Anesth Analg 1990;71:362.
51. Spear RM, Yaster M, Berkowitz ID, et al. Preinduction of anesthesia in children with rectally administered midazolam. Anesthesiology 1991;74:670.
52. Diem K, Lentner C. Scientific Tables (7th ed). Basel, Switzerland: Ciba-Geigy, 1970;635.

53. Yaster M, Maxwell LG. Pediatric regional anesthesia. Anesthesiology 1989;70:324.
54. Pennant JH, White PF. The laryngeal mask airway. Anesthesiology 1993;79:144–163.
55. Vaughan RS. Potassium in the perioperative period. Br J Anaesth 1991;67:194.
56. Parbrook GD, Davis PD, Parbrook EO. Basic Physics and Measurement in Anaesthesia. Oxford, UK: Butterworth–Heinemann, 1990;68.
57. Krane EJ, Domino KB. Anesthesia for Neurosurgery. In EK Motoyama, PJ Davis (eds), Anesthesia for Infants and Children. St. Louis: Mosby, 1990;555.
58. Bell C, Kain ZN, Hughes C. Fluids, Electrolytes, and Transfusion Therapy. In C Bell, ZN Kain, C Hughes (eds), The Pediatric Anesthesia Handbook. St. Louis: Mosby–Year Book, 1997;74.
59. Transfusion Service Manual. Durham, NC: Duke University Medical Center, 1997;55.
60. Halevy JD. Malignant Hyperthermia. In C Bell, CW Hughes, TH Oh (eds), The Pediatric Handbook. St. Louis: Mosby–Year Book, 1991;537.
61. McQuillan PJ, Morgan BA, Ramwell J. Adriamycin cardiomyopathy: fatal outcome of general anaesthesia in a child with adriamycin cardiomyopathy. Anaesthesia 1988;43:301.
62. McGoldrick K. Anesthesia for Ophthalmic Surgery. In EK Motoyama, PJ Davis (eds), Smith's Anesthesia for Infants and Children. St. Louis: Mosby–Year Book, 1990;631.
63. Bridenbaugh PO, Greene NM. Spinal (Subarachnoid) Blockade. In MJ Cousins, PO Bridenbaugh, P Madelpha (eds), Clinica! Anesthesia and Management of Pain. Philadelphia: Lippincott, 1980;213–248.
64. Dubois D, Dubois EF. Estimation of human body surface area from height and weight. Proc Soc Exp Biol Med 1916;13:17.
65. Geghan EA, George SL. A height-weight formula to estimate the surface area of man. Cancer Chemother Rep 1970;54:225.
66. Litman RS, Keon TP, Campbell FW, et al. Termination of supraventricular tachycardia with adenosine in a healthy child undergoing anesthesia. Anesth Analg 1991;73:665.
67. Buchholz DH. Blood transfusion: merits of component therapy. Part I. J Pediatr 1974;841:4.

68. Buchholz DH. Blood transfusion: merits of component therapy. Part II. The clinical use of plasma and plasma components. J Pediatr 1974;841:165.
69. Schmidt PJ. Component therapy in techniques of blood transfusion. Int Anesthesiol Clin 1982;20:23.
70. Transfusion Service Manual. Durham, NC: Duke University Medical Center, 1997;23.
71. Miller RD, Savarese JJ. Pharmacology of Muscle Relaxants and Their Antagonists. In RD Miller (ed), Anesthesia (3rd ed). New York: Churchill Livingstone, 1990;9.
72. Park MK, Lee DH. Normative arm and calf blood pressure values in the newborn. Pediatrics 1989;83:240.
73. Berry FA. Anesthetic Management of Difficult and Routine Pediatric Patients. New York: Churchill Livingstone, 1986;435.
74. Chow AE, Noble-Jamieson C. Termination of supraventricular tachycardia by IV adenosine in a child. Anaesthesia 1989;44:322.
75. Welborn LG, de Soto H, Hannallah RS, et al. The use of caffeine in the control of postanesthetic apnea in former premature infants. Anesthesiology 1988;8:796.
76. Garson A Jr. Dysrhythmias. In TF Yeh (ed), Drug Therapy in the Infant and Small Neonate. Chicago: Year Book, 1985;176.
77. Aranda JV, Gorman W, Bergensteinsson H, Gunn T. Efficacy of caffeine in the treatment of apnea in the low birth weight infant. J Pediatr 1977;90:467.
78. Pagliaro LA, Pagliaro AM. Problems in Pediatric Drug Therapy. Hamilton, IL: Drug Intelligence Publications, 1995;768.
79. Krane EJ, Domino KB. Anesthesia for Neurosurgery. In EK Motoyama, PJ Davis (eds), Smith's Anesthesia for Infants and Children. St. Louis: Mosby–Year Book, 1990;555–590.
80. Spear RM, Deshpandle JK, Davis PJ. Systemic Disorders in Pediatric Anesthesia. In EK Motoyama, PJ Davis (eds), Smith's Anesthesia for Infants and Children. St. Louis: Mosby–Year Book, 1990;788.
81. Pollard BJ, Harrison MJ. Anaesthesia for Uncommon Diseases. Oxford, UK: Blackwell, 1989;167–168.
82. McGoldrick KE. Anesthesia for Ophthalmic Surgery. In EK Motoyama, PJ Davis (eds), Smith's Anesthesia for Infants and Children. St. Louis: Mosby–Year Book, 1990;631.

83. Motoyama EK. Anesthesia for Ear, Nose, and Throat Surgery. In EK Motoyama, PJ Davis (eds), Smith's Anesthesia for Infants and Children. St. Louis: Mosby–Year Book, 1990;664.
84. Sandhar BK, Goresky GV, Maltby JR, Shaffer EA. Effect of oral liquids and ranitidine on gastric fluid volume and pH in children undergoing outpatient surgery. Anesthesiology 1989;71:327.
85. Michael RS, Barker I, Henderson P, et al. Pharmacokinetics of lidocaine in children after infiltration for cleft palate surgery. Br J Anaesth 1992;69:577.
86. Motoyama EK. Maintenance of Anesthesia. In EK Motoyama, PJ Davis (eds), Smith's Anesthesia for Infants and Children. St. Louis: Mosby–Year Book, 1990;295.
87. Wolf AR, Valley RD, Fear DW, et al. Bupivacaine for caudal analgesia in infants and children: the optimal effective concentration. Anesthesiology 1988;69:102.
88. Goudsouzian NG, Alifmoff JK, Liu LM, et al. Neuromuscular and cardiovascular effects of doxacurium in children anaesthetized with halothane. Br J Anaesth 1989;62:263.
89. Christensen S, Farrow-Gillespie A, Lehrman J. Effects of ranitidine and metoclopramide on gastric fluid pH and volume in children. Br J Anaesth 1990;65:456.
90. van Erdewyk JM. Postoperative Nausea and Vomiting. In RF Cuccharia, LH Milder, SH Rose, et al. (eds), Anesthesiology Review. New York: Churchill Livingstone, 1991;487–488.
91. Shannon M, Albers G, Burkhart K, et al. Safety and efficacy of flumazenil in the reversal of benzodiazepine-induced conscious sedation. The Flumazenil Pediatric Study Group. J Pediatr 1997;131:582–586.
92. Lowe EE. Postoperative Cardiac Care. In CL Lake (ed), Pediatric Cardiac Anesthesia. Norwalk, CT: Appleton & Lange, 1997;565.
93. Brandom BW, Carroll JB, Rosenberg H. Malignant Hyperthermia. In EK Motoyama, PJ Davis (eds), Smith's Anesthesia for Infants and Children. St. Louis: Mosby–Year Book, 1990;769.
94. Camboulives J. Indications, Effects, and Monitoring. In BJ Dalens (ed), Pediatric Regional Anesthesia. Boca Raton, FL: CRC Press, 1990;157.
95. Cohen DE, Steven JM. Anesthesia for Orthopedic Surgery. In EK Motoyama, PJ Davis (eds), Smith's Anesthesia for Infants and Children. St. Louis: Mosby–Year Book, 1990;619.

96. Berde C, Albin A, Glazer J, et al. The American Academy of Pediatrics report of the Subcommittee on Disease-Related Pain in Childhood Cancer. Pediatrics 1990;86:818.
97. Tatman AJ, Wrigley SR, Jones RM. Resistance to atracurium in a patient with increase in $alpha_1$ globulins. Br J Anaesth 1991;67:623.
98. Information from the Pharmacy Department, Duke University Medical Center, Durham, NC.
99. Strain JD, Harvey LA, Foley FC, Campbell JB. Intravenously administered pentobarbital sodium for sedation in pediatric CT. Radiology 1986;161:105.
100. Birmingham PK, Hall SC. Drug Infusions in Pediatric Anesthesia. In RJ Fragen (ed), Drug Infusions in Anesthesiology. Philadelphia: Lippincott–Raven, 1996;193–224.
101. Feld LH, Negus JB, White PF. Oral midazolam preanesthetic medication in pediatric outpatients. Anesthesiology 1990;73:831.
102. Meakin G, McKiernan EP, Morris P, Baker RD. Dose-response curves for suxamethonium in neonates, infants and children. Br J Anaesth 1989;62:655.
103. Miller JD, Rosenbaum H. Muscle Diseases. In JI Benumof (ed), Anesthesia and Uncommon Diseases. Philadelphia: Saunders, 1998;316–317.
104. Taylor RH, Lerman J. Minimum alveolar concentration of desflurane and hemodynamic responses in neonates, infants, and children. Anesthesiology 1991;75:975.
105. Koren G, Butt W, Chinyanga H, et al. Postoperative morphine infusion in newborn infants: assessment of disposition characteristics and safety. J Pediatr 1985;107:963.
106. Olkkola KT, Maunuksela EL. The pharmacokinetics of postoperative intravenous ketorolac tromethamine in children. Br J Clin Pharmacol 1991;31:182.
107. Gouveia MA. The central nervous system. Rev Braz Anesth 1970;20:501.
108. Sarner JB, Brandom BW, Woelfel SK, et al. Clinical pharmacology of mivacurium chloride (BW B1090U) in children during nitrous oxide–halothane and nitrous oxide–narcotic anesthesia. Anesth Analg 1989;68:116.
109. Brandom BW, Carroll JB, Rosenberg H. Malignant Hyperthermia. In EK Motoyama, PJ Davis (eds), Smith's Anesthesia for Infants and Children. St. Louis: Mosby–Year Book, 1990;771.

110. An Outline of Antibiotics Used at Duke Medical Center, Department of Pediatrics, 1996.
111. Patteson SK, Chesney JT. Anesthetic management for magnetic resonance imaging: problems and solutions. Anesth Analg 1992;(74):121.
112. Katoh T, Ikeda K. Minimum alveolar concentration of sevoflurane in children. Br J Anaesth 1992;68:139.
113. Murray DJ, Metha MP, Forbes, et al. The additive contribution of nitrous oxide to isoflurane MAC in infants and children. Anesthesiology 1991;75:186.
114. Claes Y, van Hemelrijck J, van Geveren M, et al. Influence of hydroxyethyl starch on coagulation in patients during the perioperative period. Anesth Analg 1992;75:24.
115. Bell CB, Hughes CW, Oh TH. The Pediatric Anesthesia Handbook. St. Louis: Mosby–Year Book, 1991;557.
116. Woelful SK, Brandom CW, Cook DR, et al. Effect of bolus administration of ORG-9426 in children during nitrous oxide-halothane anesthesia. Anesthesiology 1992;76:939–942.
117. Fisher DM, Zwass MS. MAC of desflurane in 60% nitrous oxide in infants and children. Anesthesiology 1992;76:354.
118. Johnson KB. The Harriet Lane Handbook (13th ed). St. Louis: Mosby–Year Book, 1993;363–561.
119. Palmisano BW, Setlock MA, Brown MP, et al. Dose response for atropine and heart rate in infants and children anesthetized with halothane and nitrous oxide. Anesthesiology 1991;75:238.
120. Savarese AM, Zucker HA. The Pediatric Pulmonary System. In CB Bell, CW Hughes, TH Oh (eds), The Pediatric Anesthesia Handbook. St. Louis: Mosby–Year Book, 1991;154–196.
121. Gutstein HB, Johnson KL, Heard MB, Gregory GA. Oral ketamine pre-anesthetic medication in children. Anesthesiology 1992;76:28.
122. Motoyama EK. Maintenance of Anesthesia. In EK Motoyama, PJ Davis (eds), Smith's Anesthesia for Infants and Children. St. Louis: Mosby–Year Book, 1990;298.
123. Kraus GB, Braun GG, Gotz H, et al. Famotidine dosage in children. The effect of different doses on the pH and volume of the gastric fluid. Anaesthetist 1990;39:587.
124. Brazier JL, Renaud H, Ribon B, Salle BL. Plasma xanthine levels in low birth weight infants treated or not treated with theophylline. Arch Dis Child 1979;54:194.

125. Aranda JV, Cook CE, Gorman W, et al. Pharmacologic profile of caffeine in the premature newborn infant with apnea. J Pediatr 1979;94:663.
126. Barash PG, Cullen BJ, Stoelting K. Pediatric Anesthesia. In PG Barash, BJ Cullen, K Stoelting (eds), Handbook of Clinical Anesthesia. Philadelphia: Lippincott, 1991;368.
127. Fisher DM, Canfell PC, Spellman MJ, Miller RD. Pharmacokinetics and pharmacodynamics of atracurium in infants and children. Anesthesiology 1990;73:33.
128. Ashburn MA, Streisand JB. Oral transmuscosal fentanyl: help or hindrance? Drug Safety 1994;11:295–298.
129. Frankville DD, Spear RM, Dyck JB. The dose of propofol required to prevent children from moving during magnetic resonance imaging. Anesthesiology 1993;79:953.
130. Litman RS, Wu CL, Christopher L, et al. Ondansetron decreases emesis after tonsillectomy in children. Anesth Analg 1994:78:478.
131. Manufacturer's recommendations.
132. Bevan DR, Donati F, Kopman AT. Reversal of neuromuscular blockade. Anesthesiology 1992;77:785.
133. Stanley TH, Schafer PG. Developments in Critical Care Medicine and Anesthesiology: Pediatric and Obstetrical Anesthesia. Dordrecht, The Netherlands: Kluwer, 1995;266–286.
134. Stehling L, Zauder H. Acute normovolemic hemodilution. Transfusion 1991;31:857.
135. Lehrman J, Sikich N, Kleinman S, et al. The pharmacology of sevoflurane in infants and children. Anesthesiology 1994;80:814.
136. Haberkern CM, Coles PG, Morray JP, et al. Intraoperative hypertension during surgical excision of neuroblastoma. Anesth Analg 1992;75:854.
137. Kahlil SN, Berry JM, Howard MS, et al. The antiemetic effect of lorazepam after outpatient strabismus surgery in children. Anesthesiology 1992;77:915.
138. Lanier WL, Warner DO. Intracranial elastance versus intracranial compliance: terminology should agree with that of other disciplines. Anesthesiology 1992;77:403.
139. Bell C, Hughes CW, Oh TH. The Pediatric Anesthesia Handbook. St. Louis: Mosby–Year Book, 1991;555.
140. van Hemelrijk J, Gonzales LM, White PF. Pharmacology of Intravenous Agents. In MC Rogers, JH Tinker, BG Covino, DE Long-

necker (eds), Principles and Practice of Anesthesiology. St. Louis: Mosby–Year Book, 1993;1131–1154.

141. Basta SJ. Pharmacology of Neuromuscular Drugs. In MC Rogers, JH Tinker, BG Covino, DE Longnecker (eds), Principles and Practice of Anesthesiology. St. Louis: Mosby–Year Book, 1993; 1518–1540.
142. Pusch F, Wilding E, Grabner CM. Principles in perioperative paediatric medicine. Anaesthesia 1998;53(suppl 2):69–71.
143. Peutrell LM. General Aspects. In JM Peutrell, SJ Mather (eds), Regional Anaesthesia for Babies and Children. Oxford, UK: Oxford University Press, 1997;24.
144. Lake CL. Pediatric Cardiac Anesthesia. East Norwalk, CT: Appleton & Lange, 1993;103.
145. American Society of Anesthesiologists Task Force on Blood Component Therapy. Practice guidelines for blood component therapy. Anesthesiology 1996;84:732–747.
146. Wolf AR, Hughes D. Pain relief for infants undergoing abdominal surgery: comparison of infusions of IV morphine and extradural bupivacaine. Br J Anaesth 1993;70:10.
147. American Heart Association. Resuscitation of Infants and Children. In Textbook of Advanced Cardiac Life Support (2nd ed). Dallas: American Heart Association, 1990;265.
148. Harmon WE. Fluid and Electrolytes. In JW Graef (ed), Manual of Pediatric Therapeutics (4th ed). Boston: Little, Brown, 1992;72.
149. Jabs K, Baum M. Renal Disorders. In JW Graef (ed), Manual of Pediatric Therapeutics (6th ed). Boston: Little, Brown, 1997;300.
150. Walsh EP. Formulary. In JW Graef (ed), Manual of Pediatric Therapeutics (6th ed). Boston: Little, Brown, 1997;592.
151. Cote CJ, Drop LJ, Hoaglin DC, et al. Ionized hypocalcemia after fresh-frozen plasma administration to thermally injured children: effects of infusion rate, duration, and treatment with calcium chloride. Anesth Analg 1988;67:152.
152. Casey WF, Rice LJ, Hannallah RS, et al. A comparison between bupivacaine instillation versus ilioinguinal/iliohypogastric nerve block for postoperative analgesia following inguinal herniorrhaphy in children. Anesthesiology 1990;72:637.
153. Maxwell LG, Yaster M, Wetzel RC. Penile nerve block reduces the physiological stress in newborn circumcision. Anesthesiology 1986;65:A428.

154. Sethna NF, Berde CB. Pediatric Regional Anesthesia. In GA Gregory (ed), Pediatric Anesthesia (3rd ed). New York: Churchill Livingstone, 1994;284.
155. Badgwell MJ. Anesthetic considerations for major pediatric trauma. Annual American Society of Anesthesiologists Refresher Courses. Park Ridge, IL: American Society of Anesthesiologists, 1992. Lecture #174,5.
156. Fosberg M, Wolfe LC. Blood Disorders. In JW Graef (ed), Manual of Pediatric Therapeutics (6th ed). Boston: Little, Brown, 1988;450.
157. Wolsdorf JI, Muglia L. Endocrine Disorders. In JW Graef (ed), Manual of Pediatric Therapeutics (6th ed). Philadelphia: Lippincott–Raven, 1997; 407.
158. Sessler D. Personal communication, 1991.
159. Bloch EC, Ossey KD, Ginsberg B. Tracheal intubation in children: a new method for assuring correct depth of tube placement. Anesth Analg 1988;67:590.
160. Bloch EC, Ginsberg B, Binner RJ Jr. The esophageal temperature gradient in anesthetized children. J Clin Monit Comput 1993;9:73.
161. Nadas AS, Fyler DC. Cardiac Catheterization. In AS Nadas, DC Fyler (eds), Pediatric Cardiology (1st ed). Philadelphia: Saunders, 1972;126.
162. Berkow R, Fletcher AJ. Disturbances in Newborns and Infants. In R Berkow, AJ Fletcher (eds), The Merck Manual. Rahway, NJ: Merck Research Laboratories, 1992;2003.
163. Levin R. Appendix 1: Drugs. In HW Taeusch, RA Ballard (eds), Avery's Diseases of the Newborn. Philadelphia: Saunders, 1998;1343–1348.
164. Todres ID. Asthma and Status Asthmaticus. In RA Katz (ed), Seminars in Anesthesia. Part II. Orlando, FL: Grune & Stratton, 1984;102.
165. Kaplan RF, Graves SA. Anatomic and Physiologic Differences in Infants and Children. In RA Katz (ed), Seminars in Anesthesia. Part I. Orlando, FL: Grune & Stratton, 1984;6.
166. O'Rourke PP, Crone RK. Pulmonary Physiology. In GA Gregory (ed), Pediatric Anesthesia (2nd ed). New York: Churchill Livingstone, 1989;848.
167. Rothstein P. ASA Refresher Courses in Anesthesiology. Park Ridge, IL: American Society of Anesthesiologists, 1980;8:155.
168. Splinter WM, Baxter M, MacNeill HB, et al. Oral ondansetron decreases vomiting after tonsillectomy in children. Can J Anaesth 1995;42:277–280.

169. Parbrook GD, Davis PD, Parbrook EO. Fluid Flow in Basic Physics and Measurement in Anaesthesia. Oxford, UK: Butterworth–Heinemann, 1990;69.
170. Eger EI, Saidman J, Brandstater B. Minimum alveolar anesthetic gas concentration: a standard of anesthetic potency. Anesthesiology 1965;26:756.
171. Abbott TR. Paediatric Cardiovascular Anaesthesia. In DJ Steward (ed), Some Aspects of Paediatric Anaesthesia. Amsterdam: Elsevier/North Holland Biomedical, 1982;189.
172. Berkow R, Fletcher AJ. Monitoring Drug Treatment. In R Berkow, AJ Fletcher (eds), The Merck Manual. Rahway, NJ: Merck Research Laboratories, 1992;2621.
173. Standards for Basic Intraoperative Monitoring. In Directory of Members, American Society of Anesthesiologists. Park Ridge, IL: American Society of Anesthesiologists, 1992;675.
174. Parbrook GD, Davis PD, Parbrook EO. Fluid Flow in Basic Physics and Measurement in Anaesthesia. Oxford, UK: Butterworth–Heinemann, 1990;17.
175. Cook DR, Davis PJ. Pediatric Anesthesia Pharmacology. In CL Lake (ed), Pediatric Cardiac Anesthesia. Norwalk, CT: Appleton & Lange, 1993;134.
176. American Heart Association. Standards and Guidelines for cardiopulmonary resuscitation (CPR) and emergency cardiac care (ECC). National Academy of Sciences—National Research Council. JAMA 1986;255:2954.
177. Grunwald Z, Torjman M, Schieren H, Bartowski RR. The pharmacokinetics of droperidol in anesthetized children. Anesth Analg 1993;76:1238.
178. Cashman JN. Nonsteroidal anti-inflammatory drugs versus postoperative pain. J Royal Soc Med 1993;86:464.
179. Goetting MG, Paradis NA. High-dose epinephrine improves outcome from pediatric cardiac arrest. Ann Emerg Med 1991;20:22.
180. Transfusion Service Manual. Durham, NC: Duke University Medical Center, 1997;38.
181. Weir PM, Munro HM, Reynolds PI, et al. Propofol infusion and the incidence of emesis in pediatric outpatient strabismus surgery. Anesth Analg 1993;76:760.
182. Haberkern CM, Mulroy JJ. Liver Diseases. In FA Berry, DJ Steward (eds), Pediatrics for the Anesthesiologist. New York: Churchill Livingstone, 1993;146.

183. Rogers PCJ, Wadsworth LD. Hematology and Oncology. In FA Berry, DJ Steward (eds), Pediatrics for the Anesthesiologist. New York: Churchill Livingstone, 1993;79.
184. McNichol R. Postoperative analgesia in children using continuous S.C. morphine. Br J Anaesth 1993;71:752.
185. Cook DR, Rowe MI. Parenteral Fluid Therapy. In DR Cook, JH Marcy (eds), Neonatal Anesthesia. Pasadena, CA: Appleton Davies, 1988;76.
186. Stack A, McManus M, Krauss B. Emergency and Intensive Care. In JW Graef (ed), Manual of Pediatric Therapeutics (6th ed). Boston: Little, Brown, 1997;224.
187. Melgrave AP. The use of epinephrine in the presence of halothane in children. Can J Anaesth 1970;17:256.
188. Karl HW, Swerdlow DB, Lee KW, et al. Epinephrine/halothane interactions in children. Anesthesiology 1983;58:142.
189. Ueda W, Hirakawa M, Mae O. Appraisal of epinephrine administration to patients under halothane anesthesia for closure of cleft palate. Anesthesiology 1983;58:574.
190. Berde C. Bupivacaine toxicity secondary to continuous caudal infusion in children. Anesth Analg 1993;77:1305.
191. Motoyama EK, Davis PJ. An Index of Syndromes and Their Anesthetic Implications. In EK Motoyama, PJ Davis (eds), Smith's Anesthesia for Infants and Children. St. Louis: Mosby–Year Book, 1990;892.
192. Young GJ, Priebe CJ. Formulary. In JW Graef (ed), Manual of Pediatric Therapeutics (6th ed). Boston: Little, Brown, 1997;574.
193. Hamunen EL. Pharmacokinetics of IV and rectal pethidine in children undergoing ophthalmic surgery. Br J Anaesth 1993;71:823.
194. Goudsouzian NG, Denman W, Schwartz A, et al. Pharmacodynamic and hemodynamic effects of mivacurium in infants anesthetized with halothane and nitrous oxide. Anesthesiology 1993;79:919.
195. Nelson JD. Pocketbook of Pediatric Antimicrobial Therapy. Baltimore: Williams & Wilkins, 1993;16–17.
196. Broadman LM, Rice LJ. Neural Blockade for Pediatric Surgery. In MJ Cousins, PO Bridenbaugh (eds), Neural Blockade in Clinical Anesthesia and Management of Pain. Philadelphia: Lippincott, 1998;615–637.
197. Gregg N, Wall C, Green D. Humidification reduces coughing and breath-holding during inhalation induction with isoflurane in children. Can J Anaesth 1996;43:1090–1094.

198. Maxwell LG, Martin LD, Yaster M. Bupivacaine-induced cardiac toxicity in neonates: successful treatment with intravenous phenytoin. Anesthesiology 1994;80:682.
199. Motoyama EK. Respiratory Physiology in Infants and Children. In EK Motoyama, PJ Davis (eds), Smith's Anesthesia for Infants and Children. St. Louis: Mosby–Year Book, 1990;26.
200. Graf G, Rosenbaum S. Anesthesia and the Endocrine System. In PG Barash, BF Cullen, RK Stoelting (eds), Clinical Anesthesia. Philadelphia: Lippincott, 1992;1251.
201. Hackel A. Preoperative Evaluation. In GA Gregory (ed), Pediatric Anesthesia. New York: Churchill Livingstone, 1983;415.
202. Transfusion Service Manual. Durham, NC: Duke University Medical Center, 1997;62.
203. Young GJ, Priebe CJ. Formulary. In JW Graef (ed), Manual of Pediatric Therapeutics (6th ed). Boston: Little, Brown, 1997;563–603.
204. Marshall BE, Longnecker DE. General Anesthetics. In AG Gilman, TW Rall, AS Nies, P Taylor (eds), The Pharmacological Basis of Therapeutics. New York: Pergamon, 1990;301.
205. Quaynor H, Corbey M, Bjorkman S. Rectal induction of anaesthesia in children with methohexitone. Br J Anaesth 1985;57:573.
206. Mitchell AA, Louik C, Lacouture P, et al. Risks to children from computed tomographic scan premedication. JAMA 1982;247:2385–2388.
207. Jamali S, Monin S, Begon D, et al. Clonidine in pediatric anesthesia. Anesth Analg 1994;78:663.
208. Broadman LM, Hannalah MS, Balman AB. Postcircumcision analgesia—a prospective evaluation of ring block of the penis. Anaesthesiology 1987;67:399.
209. Parbrook GD, Davis PD, Parbrook EO. Pressure. Basic Physics and Measurement in Anaesthesia.(4th ed). Oxford, UK: Butterworth–Heinemann, 1995;1.
210. Motoyama EK, Davis PJ. Anesthesia for Trauma. In EK Motoyama, PJ Davis (eds), Smith's Anesthesia for Infants and Children (6th ed). St. Louis: Mosby–Year Book, 1996;794.
211. Lowe EL. Postoperative Cardiac Care. In CL Lake (ed), Pediatric Cardiac Anesthesia. Norwalk, CT: Appleton & Lange, 1997;547–576.
212. Rheuban KS, Carpenter MA. Diagnostic Cardiac Catheterization, Angiography, and Interventional Catheterization. In CL Lake (ed), Pediatric Cardiac Anesthesia. Norwalk, CT: Appleton & Lange, 1997;73.

213. Mikawa A, Maekawa N, Takao Y, et al. Efficacy of oral premedication in children. Anesthesiology 1992;77:A1169.
214. Lerman J. Special techniques: Acute Normovolemic Hemodilution, Controlled Hypotension, and Controlled Hypothermia. In GA Gregory (ed), Pediatric Anesthesia (2nd ed). New York: Churchill Livingstone, 1989;783.
215. Levy JH. Anaphylactic Reactions in Anesthesia and Intensive Care (2nd ed). Boston: Butterworth–Heinemann, 1992;136–162.
216. Lye MA, Jamieson JW. Blood pressure measurement using finger cuffs: comparison with arm cuffs during general anaesthesia in children and young adults. Anaesthesia 1994;49:895–899.
217. Hatch D, Sumner E, Hellman J. The Adrenergic Effect of Catecholamines. In D Hatch, E Sumner, J Hellman (eds), The Surgical Neonate: Anaesthesia and Intensive Care. London: Edward Arnold, 1995;239.
218. Hatch D, Sumner E, Hellman J. Acute Treatment of Supraventricular Tachycardia. In D Hatch, E Sumner, J Hellman (eds), The Surgical Neonate: Anaesthesia and Intensive Care. London: Edward Arnold, 1995;242.
219. Hatch D, Sumner E, Hellman J. Perinatal Physiology and Medicine. In D Hatch, E Sumner, J Hellman (eds), The Surgical Neonate: Anaesthesia and Intensive Care. London: Edward Arnold, 1995;69.
220. Ray S, Rubin P. Anaesthesia in a child with Schwartz-Jampel syndrome. Anaesthesia 1994;49:600–602.
221. Critchley LAH, Gin T, Stuart JC. Anaesthesia for an infant with Rubenstein-Taybi syndrome. Anaesthesia 1995;50:37–38.
222. Jagtap SR, Malde AD, Pantviadya SH. Anesthetic considerations in a patient with Fraser syndrome. Anaesthesia 1995;50:39–41.
223. Karl HW, Rosenberger JL, Larch MG, et al. Transmucosal administration of midazolam for premedication in pediatric patients. Anesthesiology 1993;78:885–891.
224. Maekwana K, Maekwana N, Nishiana K, et al. Efficacy of oral clonidine premedication in children. Anaesthesiology 1993;79:926–941.
225. Lonnqvist PA, Bergendahl HTG, Eksborg S. Pharmacokinetics of clonidine after rectal administration in children. Anesthesiology 1994;81:1097–1101.
226. Vuksanaj D, Fisher DM. Pharmacokinetics in children aged 4–11 years. Anesthesiology 1995;82:1104–1110.

227. Weksler N, Ovidia L, Muati G, et al. Nasal ketamine for paediatric premedication. Can J Anaesth 1993;40:119–121.
228. Rice LJ. Regional Anesthesia in the Pediatric Patient. In TH Stanley, PG Schafer (eds), Developments in Critical Care Medicine and Anesthesiology: Pediatric and Obstetrical Anesthesia. Dordrecht, The Netherlands: Kluwer, 1995;300.
229. Jerman J. Postoperative Nausea and Vomiting in Children. In TH Stanley, PG Schafer (eds), Developments in Critical Care Medicine and Anesthesiology: Pediatric and Obstetrical Anesthesia. Dordrecht, The Netherlands: Kluwer, 1995;303–314.
230. Fink JB, Jue PK. Humidity and Aerosol Therapy for Pediatrics. In SL Barnhart, MP Czervinske (eds), Perinatal and Pediatric Respiratory Care. Philadelphia: Saunders, 1995;181.
231. Smith L. Childhood asthma: diagnosis and treatment. Curr Probl Pediatr 1993;23:271–305.
232. Allen ED, McCoy KS. Airway Disorders. In SL Barnhart, MP Czervinske (eds), Perinatal and Pediatric Respiratory Care. Philadelphia: Saunders, 1995;497.
233. Ghajar J, Hariri RJ. Management of pediatric head injury. Pediatr Clin North Am 1992;39:1107.
234. Jaffe R. Reproduced with written kind permission of the compiler, Rory Jaffe, MD.
235. Maunuksela EL, Ryhanen P, Lanhunen L. Efficacy of rectal ibuprofen in controlling postoperative pain in children. Can J Anaesth 1992;39:226–230.
236. Carbajal R, Simon N, Blanc P, et al. Rectal flumazenil to reverse midazolam sedation in children. Can J Anaesth 1996;83:895.
237. McLoughlin CC, Mirakhur RK. Muscle Relaxants in Paediatric Anaesthesia. In NJN Harper, BJ Pollard (eds), Muscle Relaxants in Anaesthesia. London: Edward Arnold, 1995;211.
238. Woolf PK. The Pediatric Electrocardiogram. In MH Gewitz (ed), Primary Pediatric Cardiology. Armonk, NY: Futura, 1995; 81–99.
239. Rylance GW. Textbook of Neonatology. London: Churchill Livingstone, 1992;1193–1211.
240. Clark JR, Smith LJ, Kendall BE, et al. Unexplained brainstem compression following routine surgery in a child with oto-palato-digital syndrome. Anaesthesia 1995;50:641–643.

241. Gall CG Jr, Stern AM, Pognanski AW, et al. Oro-palato-digital syndrome: comparison of clinical and radiographic manifestations in males and females. Am J Hum Genet 1972;24:24–36.
242. Bell C, Kain ZN. Acute Pediatric Pain Management. In C Bell, ZN Kain (eds), The Pediatric Handbook. St. Louis: Mosby–Year Book 1997;459.
243. Gadiyar V, Gallagher TM, Crean PM, et al. The effect of a combination of rectal diclofenac and caudal bupivacaine on postoperative analgesia in children. Anaesthesia 1995;50:820–822.
244. Ray PJ. Acute Pain Syndromes in Children. In PJ Ray (ed), Pain Medicine: A Comprehensive Review. St. Louis: Mosby–Year Book, 1996;530–536.
245. Henderson JM. Preinduction of anesthesia in pediatric patients with nasally administered sufentanil. Anesthesiology, 1996;68: 671–675.
246. Cornblath M, Schwartz R, Aynsley-Green A, et al. Hypoglycemia in infants: the need for a rational definition. Pediatrics 1990;85:834–837.
247. Taketomo CK, Hodding JH, Kraus DM. Pediatric Dosage Handbook. Hudson, OH: Lexi-Corp, 1996;19–720.
248. Barash PG, Cullen BJ, Stoelting K. Pediatric Anesthesia. In PG Barash, BJ Cullen, K Stoelting (eds), Handbook of Clinical Anesthesia. Philadelphia: Lippincott, 1991;480.
249. McLoughlin CC, Mirakhur RK. Muscle Relaxants in Paediatric Anaesthesia. In NJN Harper, BJ Pollard (eds), Muscle Relaxants in Anaesthesia. London: Edward Arnold, 1995;204.
250. Stack A, McManus M, Krauss B. Emergency and Intensive Care. In JW Graef (ed), Manual of Pediatric Therapeutics (6th ed). Boston: Little, Brown, 1997;224.
251. Bell C, Kain ZN. Respiratory Physiology and Disease Processes. In C Bell, ZN Kain (eds), The Pediatric Handbook. St. Louis: Mosby–Year Book, 1997;123.
252. Bell C, Kain ZN. Anesthesia for Otolaryngoloic Surgery. In C Bell, ZN Kain (eds), The Pediatric Handbook. St. Louis: Mosby–Year Book, 1997;198.
253. Bell C, Kain ZN. Anesthesia for Gastrointestinal Disorders. In C Bell, ZN Kain (eds), The Pediatric Handbook. St. Louis: Mosby–Year Book, 1997;247.
254. Andrew M, Paes B, Milner R, et al. The development of the human coagulation system in the full term infant. Blood 1987;70:165–172.

255. Bell C, Kain ZN. Children with Endocrine Dysfunction. In C Bell, ZN Kain (eds), The Pediatric Handbook. St. Louis: Mosby–Year Book, 1997;318–319.
256. Bell C, Kain ZN. Premedication. In C Bell, ZN Kain (eds), The Pediatric Handbook. St. Louis: Mosby–Year Book, 1997;30.
257. Taketomo CK, Hodding JH, Kraus DM. Pediatric Dosage Handbook. Hudson, OH: Lexi-Corp, 1996;542.
258. Taketomo CK, Hodding JH, Kraus DM. Pediatric Dosage Handbook. Hudson, OH: Lexi-Corp, 1996;29.
259. Reynolds L. Useful Drugs in the Operative Period. In GA Gregory (ed), Pediatric Anesthesia (3rd ed). New York: Churchill Livingstone, 1994;901–904.
260. Pagliaro LA, Pagliaro AM. Problems in Pediatric Drug Therapy. Hamilton, IL: Drug Intelligence Publications, 1995;995.
261. Taketomo CK, Hodding JH, Kraus DM. Pediatric Dosage Handbook. Hudson, OH: Lexi-Corp, 1996;177.
262. Bell C, Kain ZN. Premedication. In C Bell, ZN Kain (eds), The Pediatric Handbook. St. Louis: Mosby–Year Book, 1997;439.
263. Taketomo CK, Hodding JH, Kraus DM. Pediatric Dosage Handbook. Hudson, OH: Lexi-Corp, 1996;380.
264. Taketomo CK, Hodding JH, Kraus DM. Pediatric Dosage Handbook. Hudson, OH: Lexi-Corp, 1996;440.
265. Bell C, Kain ZN. The Pediatric Handbook. St. Louis: Mosby–Year Book, 1997;609.
266. Hollinger IB. Diseases of the Cardiovascular System. In J Katz, D Steward (eds), Anesthesia and Uncommon Pediatric Diseases. Philadelphia: Saunders, 1987;153.
267. Bell C, Kain ZN. The Pediatric Handbook. St. Louis: Mosby–Year Book, 1997;626.
268. Bell C, Kain ZN. The Pediatric Handbook St. Louis: Mosby–Year Book, 1997;607.
269. Taketomo CK, Hodding JH, Kraus DM. Pediatric Dosage Handbook. Hudson, OH: Lexi-Corp, 1996;44.
270. Bell C, Kain ZN. Appendix A. In C Bell, ZN Kain (eds), The Pediatric Handbook St. Louis: Mosby–Year Book, 1997;627.
271. Kern FH, Schulman SR, Scott-Lawson CCP, et al. Extracorporeal Circulation and Circulatory Assist Devices in the Pediatric Patient. In CL Lake (ed), Pediatric Cardiac Anesthesia. Stamford, CT: Appleton & Lange, 1997;228–229.

272. Pagliaro LA, Pagliaro AM. Drug Dosing in Infants, Children, and Adolescents. In LA Pagliaro, AM Pagliaro (eds), Problems in Pediatric Drug Therapy. Hamilton, IL: Drug Intelligence Publications, 1995;607.
273. Bell C, Kain ZN. Appendix E. In C Bell, ZN Kain (eds), The Pediatric Handbook. St. Louis: Mosby–Year Book, 1997;665.
274. Kannan S, Delph Y, Moseley HSL. Anaesthetic management of a child with Bartter's syndrome. Can J Anaesth 1995;42:808–812.
275. Taketomo CK, Hodding JH, Kraus DM. Pediatric Dosage Handbook. Hudson, OH: Lexi-Corp, 1996;369.
276. Bell C, Kain ZN. The Pediatric Handbook. St. Louis: Mosby–Year Book, 1997;462.
277. Pagliaro LA, Pagliaro AM. Problems in Pediatric Drug Therapy. Hamilton, IL: Drug Intelligence Publications, 1995;939.
278. Pagliaro LA, Pagliaro AM. Problems in Pediatric Drug Therapy. Hamilton, IL: Drug Intelligence Publications, 1995;903.
279. Hickey PR, Wessel DL. Anesthesia for Congenital Heart Disease. In GA Gregory (ed), Pediatric Anesthesia (2nd ed). New York: Churchill Livingstone, 1989;850.
280. Advanced Cardiac Life Support Working Group. In Textbook of Advanced Cardiac Life Support (2nd ed). Dallas: American Heart Association, 1992;255–256.
281. Bell C, Kain ZN. The Pediatric Anesthesia Handbook. St. Louis: Mosby–Year Book, 1997;281.
282. van Obberg LJ, Muller G, Fieppen B, et al. Propofol infusion and laryngeal mask insertion for magnetic resonance imaging in children. Anesthesiology 1992;77:177.
283. Trotter C, Serpell MG. Neurologic sequellae in children after prolonged propofol infusion. Anaesthesia 1992;47:340–343.
284. Park TJ, Stevens JE, Rice ASC, et al. Metabolic acidosis and fatal myocardial failure after propofol infusion in children. Five case reports. BMJ 1992;305:613–616.
285. Hatch D, Sumner E, Hellman J. The Surgical Neonate: Anaesthesia and Intensive Care. London: Edward Arnold, 1995;223.
286. Ostheimer GW. Resuscitation of the Newborn. In TH Stanley, PG Schafer (eds), Developments in Critical Care Medicine and Anesthesiology: Pediatric and Obstetrical Anesthesia. Dordrecht, The Netherlands: Kluwer, 1995;181.

287. Gronert BJ, Motoyama EK. Induction of Anesthesia and Endotracheal Intubation. In EK Motoyama, PJ Davis (eds), Smith's Anesthesia for Infants and Children. St. Louis: Mosby–Year Book, 1996;303.
288. Broadman LM, Rice LJ. Pediatric regional anesthesia and perioperative analgesia. Probl Anesth 1988;2:386.
289. Vener DF, Carr DS, Shich N, et al. Does diphenhydramine control vomiting in children after outpatient strabismus surgery? Anesthesiology 1994;81:A21.
290. Jones EP, Pelton DA. An index of syndromes and their anesthetic implications. Can Anaesth Soc J 1976;23:207.
291. Motoyama EK, Davis PJ. Regional Anesthesia and Analgesia. In EK Motoyama, PJ Davis (eds), Smith's Anesthesia for Infants and Children. St. Louis: Mosby–Year Book, 1996;403–442.
292. Reynolds LM, Lau M, Brown BS, et al. Intramuscular rocuronium in infants and children: dose-ranging and intubating conditions. Anesthesiology 1996;85:231–329.
293. Walker SM. Introduction to Pain in Pediatric and Neonatal Patients. In MJ Cousins, W Bridenbaugh (eds), Neural Blockade in Clinical Anesthesia and Management of Pain. Philadelphia: Lippincott–Raven, 1998;720.
294. Schwartz N, Eisenkraft JB. Probable venous air embolism during epidural placement in an infant. Anesth Analg 1993;76:1136.
295. Dohi S, Naito H, Takahashi T. Age related changes in blood pressure and duration of motor block in spinal anesthesia. Anesthesiology 1979;50:319.
296. Bell C, Kain ZN. The Pediatric Anesthesia Handbook. St. Louis: Mosby–Year Book, 1997;73.
297. Rowney DA, Doyle E. Epidural and subarachnoid blockade in children. Anaesthesia 1998;53:980–1001.
298. Karl HW, Rosenberger JL, Larach MG, et al. Transmucosal administration of midazolam for premedication in pediatric patients. Anesthesiology 1993;78:885–891.
299. Gutstein HB, Johnson KL, Heard MB, et al. Oral ketamine preanesthetic medication in children. Anesthesiology 1992;76:28–33.
300. Lerman J. New Inhalational Anesthetics in Infants and Children. In TH Stanley, PG Schafer (eds), Developments in Critical Care Medicine and Anesthesiology: Pediatric and Obstetrical Anesthesia. Dordrecht, The Netherlands: Kluwer, 1995;266–268.

301. Woolf PK. The Pediatric Electrocardiogram. In MH Gewitz (ed), Primary Pediatric Cardiology. Armonk, NY: Futura, 1995;81–99.
302. Schechter NL, Weisman SJ, Rosenblum M, et al. The use of oral transmuscosal fentanyl citrate for painful procedures in children. Pediatrics 1995;95:335–339.
303. Rylance GW. Textbook of Neonatology. London: Churchill Livingstone, 1992;1193–1211.
304. Silverman BK (ed). The Pediatric Emergency Course (2nd ed). Elk Grove Village, IL: American Academy of Pediatrics, 1993;237.
305. Dinner M, Goldin EZ, Ward R, et al. Russel-Silver syndrome: anesthetic implications. Anesth Analg 1994;78:1197–1199.
306. Rusky LM, Houck CS, Sullivan LJ, et al. A double blind evaluation of ketorolac tromethamine and acetaminophen in pediatric tonsillectomy: analgesia and bleeding. Anesth Analg 1995;80:226–229.
307. Lubinsky P. Aerosols. In HW Taeush, RO Cristiansen, ES Buescher (eds), Pediatric and Neonatal Tests and Procedures. Philadelphia: Saunders, 1996;59–65.
308. Levin HL, Fernandez SV, Luing I, et al. Management of Pain and Sedation. In HW Taeush, RO Cristiansen, ES Buescher (eds), Pediatric and Neonatal Tests and Procedures. Philadelphia: Saunders, 1996;179–196.
309. Riazi J. The Difficult Pediatric Airway. In JL Beumof (ed), Airway Management: Practice and Principles. St. Louis: Mosby–Year Book, 1996; 585–637.
310. Fujii Y, Tanaka H, Toyooka H. Granisetron reduces vomiting after strabismus surgery and tonsillectomy in children. Can J Anaesth 1996;43:35–38.
311. Tobias J, Rasmusson GE, Holcomb GW, et al. Continuous caudal anaesthesia with chloroprocaine as an adjunct to general anesthesia in neonates. Can J Anaesth 1996;43:69–72.
312. Rice LJ. Pediatric Sedation Challenges Outside the Operating Room. In MA Ashburn, PG Fine, TH Stanley (eds), Pain Management in Anesthesiology. Boston: Kluwer, 1998;205–216.
313. Cost M. Specific Patient Populations: Pediatrics. In M Cost (ed), Manual of Conscious Sedation. Philadelphia: Saunders, 1998; 152–161.
314. Stimson JM. Pharmacology. In SL Barnhart, MP Czervinske (eds), Perinatal and Pediatric Respiratory Care. Philadelphia: Saunders, 1995;418–431.

315. Gregory GA. Pharmacology. In GA Gregory (ed), Pediatric Anesthesia (3rd ed). New York: Churchill Livingstone, 1994;19.
316. Jonmarker C, Westrin P, Larsson S, et al. Thiopental requirements for induction of anesthesia in children. Anesthesiology 1987;67: 104–107.
317. Mesrobian RB. Stridor in the Recovery Room. In L Stehling (ed), Common Problems in Pediatric Anesthesia. St. Louis: Mosby–Year Book, 1992;189–195.
318. Scott JP. Hematology. In RE Behrman, RM Kliegman (eds), Nelson Essentials of Pediatrics. Philadelphia: Saunders, 1998;581.
319. Rice LJ. Regional Anesthesia Techniques. In PF White (ed), Ambulatory Anesthesia and Surgery. Philadelphia: Saunders, 1997; 583–631.
320. Dajani AS, Bisno AL, Chung KJ, et al. Prevention of Bacterial Endocarditis. Recommendations by the American Heart Association. JAMA 1990;264:2919–2922.
321. Mercsmar CM. The Respiratory System. In RE Behrman, RM Kliegman (eds), Nelson Essentials of Pediatrics. Philadelphia: Saunders, 1998;459–916.
322. Friedman AL. Nephrology: Fluids and Electrolytes. In RE Behrman, RM Kliegman (eds), Nelson Essentials of Pediatrics. Philadelphia: Saunders, 1998;609–646.
323. Painter MJ, Bergman I. Neurology. In RE Behrman, RM Kliegman (eds), Nelson Essentials of Pediatrics. Philadelphia: Saunders, 1998;694–745.
324. Behrman RE, Kliegman RM. Appendices. In RE Behrman, RM Kliegman (eds), Nelson Essentials of Pediatrics. Philadelphia: Saunders, 1998;783–801.
325. Tan CH, Onsiong MK. Pain on injection of propofol. Anaesthesia 1998;53:468–476.
326. Peutrell LM. Extradural Anaesthesia. In JM Peutrell, SJ Mather (eds), Regional Anaesthesia for Babies and Children. Oxford, UK: Oxford University Press, 1997;187–233.
327. Hatch D, Sumner E, Hellman J. The Surgical Neonate: Anaesthesia and Intensive Care. London: Edward Arnold, 1995;294.
328. Kozek-Langenecker S, Chiari A, Semsroth M. Simulation of an epidural test dose with intravenous isoprotorenol in awake and halothane-anesthetized children. Anesthesiology 1996;85: 277–280.

329. Mayhew JF, Jones R, Dolcourt J. Anesthesia for the patient with the Freeman-Sheldon syndrome. Anesthesiology 1993;78:408.
330. Kuzma PJ, Calkins MD. Multiple pterygium syndrome. Anesth Analg 1996;83:430–432.
331. Phillips S, Hatch DJ. Preoperative fasting for paediatric anaesthesia. Br J Anaesth. 1994;73:529–536.
332. Pennant JH, White P. The laryngeal mask airway: its uses in anesthesiology (review article). Anesthesiology 1993;79:144–163.
333. Bouaziz B, Laxenaire MC. Anaesthesia for the allergic patient. Curr Opin Anaesthesiol 1998;11:339–344.
334. Laxenaire MC and the "Groupe d'Etude des Reactions Anaphylactiodes Peranesthesiques." Substances responsible des chocs anaphylactiques peranesthesiques. Troisieme enquete multicentrique francaise (1992–1994). Ann Fr Anesth Reanim 1996;15:1211–1218.
335. American Academy of Pediatrics Committee on Drugs. Guidelines for monitoring and management of pediatric patients during and after sedation for diagnostic and therapeutic procedures. Pediatrics 1992;89:1110–1115.
336. Takasaki M, Dohi S, Kwabata Y, Takahashi T. Dosage of lidocaine for caudal anesthesia in infants and children. Anesthesiology 1997;47:527–529.
337. Dalens BJ. Pediatric Regional Anesthesia. Boca Raton, FL: CRC Press, 1990;424.
338. Berde C. General Approach to Pediatric Anesthesia. In EK Motoyama, PJ Davis (eds), Smith's Anesthesia for Infants and Children. St. Louis: Mosby–Year Book, 1996;394.
339. Tanaka M, Toshiaki N. Simulation of an epidural test dose with intravenous epinephrine in sevoflurane-anesthetized children. Anesth Analg 1998;86:952–957.
340. Glass PSA, Estok P, Ginsberg B, et al. Use of patient-controlled analgesia to compare the efficacy of epidural to intravenous fentanyl administration. Anesth Analg 1992;74:345–351.
341. Muir MR, Sullivan FL, Dear G, Ginsberg B. Monitoring practices following epidural analgesics for pain management: a follow-up survey. J Pain Symptom Manage 1997;14:36–44.
342. Dalens B. Intravenous Regional Anesthesia. In B Dalens (ed), Regional Anesthesia in Infants, Children and Adolescents. London: Williams-Waverly Europe, 1997;499.

343. Dalens B. Principal Techniques of Local Anesthesia. In B Dalens (ed), Regional Anesthesia in Infants, Children and Adolescents. London: Williams-Waverly Europe, 1997;507.
344. Rice LJ. Ketamine—from "Star Wars" to Dinosaur in 25 Years? In TH Stanley, PG Shafer (eds), Pediatric and Obstetrical Anesthesia. Dordrecht, The Netherlands: Kluwer, 1995;345.
345. Cravero JP, Manzi DJ, Rice LJ. The Management of Procedure-Related Pain in the Child. In MA Ashburn, LJ Rice (eds), The Management of Pain. New York: Churchill Livingstone, 1998;667–681.
346. Rita L, Frank LS, Mazurek A, et al. Intramuscular midazolam for pediatric preanesthetic sedation: a double blind controlled study with morphine. Anesthesiology 1985;63:528.
347. Tobias JD. Postoperative Pain Management. In JK Deshpanade, JD Tobias (eds), The Pediatric Pain Handbook. St. Louis: Mosby–Year Book, 1996;49–80.
348. Morray JP, Krane EJ, Geiduschek JM, et al. Anesthesia for Thoracic Surgery. In GA Gregory (ed), Pediatric Anesthesia (3rd ed). New York: Churchill Livingstone, 1994;454.
349. Mitenko PA, Ogilvie RI. Rational intravenous doses of theophylline. N Engl J Med 1973;289:600.
350. Krane EJ. Delayed respiratory depression in a child after caudal epidural morphine. Anesth Analg 1988;67:79.
351. Houck CS, Berde CB, Anand KJS. Pediatric Pain Management. In GA Gregory (ed), Pediatric Anesthesia (3rd ed). New York: Churchill Livingstone, 1994;743–771.
352. Berde CB. Convulsions associated with pediatric regional anesthesia. Anesth Analg 1992;75:164.
353. Benlabed MRD, Ecoffey C, Levin JC, et al. Analgesia and ventilatory response to CO_2 following epidural sufentanil in children. Anesthesiology 1987;67:948.
354. Houck CS. The Management of Acute Pain in the Child. In MA Ashburn, LJ Rice (eds), The Management of Pain. New York: Churchill Livingstone, 1998;651–666.
355. Dalens B, Chrysostome Y. Intervertebral epidural anaesthesia in paediatric surgery: success rate and adverse effects in 650 consecutive procedures. Paediatr Anaesth 1991;1:107–117.
356. Rash SK, Carter B. Clinical Manual of Pediatric Anesthesia. New York: McGraw-Hill, 1994.

357. Steward DJ. Preoperative Evaluation and Preparation for Surgery. In GA Gregory (ed), Pediatric Anesthesia (3rd ed). New York: Churchill Livingstone, 1994;187.
358. Perry JC, Knilans TK, Marlow D, et al. Intravenous amiodarone for life-threatening tachyarrhythmias in children and young adults. J Am Coll Cardiol 1993;22:95–98.
359. Perry JC, Enrich AL, Hulsea JE, et al. Clinical efficacy and safety of intravenous amiodarone in infants and children. Am J Cardiol 1993;74:573–577.
360. Wright JL, Patterson MD. Resuscitating the pediatric patient. Emerg Clin North Am 1996;14:219–231.
361. Fisher DM. Anesthesia Equipment for Pediatrics. In GA Gregory (ed), Pediatric Anesthesia (3rd ed). New York: Churchill Livingstone, 1994;216.
362. Cauldwell CB. Induction, Maintenance and Emergence. In GA Gregory (ed), Pediatric Anesthesia (3rd ed). New York: Churchill Livingstone, 1994;244.
363. Bosenberg AT, Bland BA, Schulte-Steinberg O, et al. Thoracic epidural anesthesia via the caudal route in infants. Anesthesiology 1988;69:265–269.
364. Hickey PR, Hansen DD, Cramolini MD. Pulmonary and systemic hemodynamic responses to ketamine in infants with normal and elevated pulmonary vascular resistance. Anesthesiology 1985;62:287.
365. Personal communication. Transfusion Service, Duke University Medical Center, Durham, NC, 1997.
366. Guidelines for red blood cell and plasma transfusion for adults and children. Expert working group. Special supplement. Can Med Assoc J 1997;156(suppl 11):59–60.
367. Meretoja OA, Meakin G, Tiavainent T, et al. Cardiovascular effects and time-course action of cisatracurium in infants and children during thiopentone-alfentanil-nitrous oxide anaesthesia. Br J Anaesth 1997;79:683–684.
368. Thompson VA, Wahr JA. Anesthetic considerations in patients with mitochondrial myopathy, encephalopathy, lactic acidosis, and stroke-like episodes (MELAS) syndrome. Anesth Analg 1997;85:1404–1406.
369. Ang C, Habre W, Sims C. Tropisetron reduces vomiting after tonsillectomy in children. Br J Anaesth 1998;80:761–763.

370. Chameides L, Brown GE, Raye JR, et al. Guidelines for defibrillation in infants and children: report of the American Heart Association Target Activity Group: cardiopulmonary resuscitation in the young. Circulation 1977;56:502A–503A.
371. Da Conceicao MJ, Coelho L. Caudal anaesthesia with 0.375% ropivacaine or 0.375% bupivacaine in pediatric patients. Br J Anaesth 1988;80:507–508.
372. Murat I. Pharmacology. In B Dalens (ed), Regional Anesthesia in Infants, Children and Adolescents. London: Williams-Waverly Europe, 1995;104–125.
373. Dalens B. Lumbar Epidural Anesthesia. In B Dalens (ed), Regional Anesthesia in Infants, Children and Adolescents. London: Williams-Waverly Europe, 1995;207–248.
374. Schulte-Steinberg O. Regional anaesthesia for children. Ann Chir Gynaecol 1984;73:158–165.
375. Saint-Maurice C. Spinal Anesthesia. In B Dalens (ed), Regional Anesthesia in Infants, Children and Adolescents. London: Williams-Waverley Europe, 1995;260–273.
376. Brink LW. Preoperative and Postoperative Care of the Newborn with Congenital Heart Disease. In HW Taeusch, RA Ballard (eds), Avery's Diseases of the Newborn. Philadelphia: Saunders, 1998;767.
377. Sessions CS. Bacterial Infections in the Newborn. In HW Taeusch, RA Ballard (eds), Avery's Diseases of the Newborn. Philadelphia: Saunders, 1998;491.
378. Savarese JJ. Interaction of Antibiotics with Muscle Relaxants, Neostigmine, and Calcium. In RD Miller (ed), Pharmacology of Muscle Relaxants and Their Antagonists in Anesthesia. New York: Churchill Livingstone, 1990;424.
379. Moore RA. Preoperative Preparation and Evaluation of the Pediatric Patient with Cardiac Disease. In CL Lake (ed), Pediatric Cardiac Anesthesia. Stamford, CT: Appleton & Lange, 1997;103.
380. Rasmussen JE. Epidural Spinal Anesthesia and Analgesia. In JK Deshpanade, JD Tobias (eds), The Pediatric Pain Handbook. St. Louis: Mosby–Year Book, 1996;84.
381. Lowe S, Hershey S. Sedation for Sedation and Imaging Procedures. In JK Deshpanade, JD Tobias (eds), The Pediatric Pain Handbook. St. Louis: Mosby–Year Book, 1996;279.

382. Reents SR, Seymour J. Clinical Pharmacology: An Electronic Reference and Teaching Guide (book on CD-rom). Tampa, FL: Gold Standard Multimedia, 1998.
383. Tobias JD. Regional Nerve Blocks and Interpleural Analgesia. In JK Deshpanade, JD Tobias (eds), The Pediatric Pain Handbook. St. Louis: Mosby–Year Book, 1996;115.
384. Broadman L. Pediatric Regional Anesthesia. In MF Mulroy (ed), Regional Anesthesia: An Illustrated Procedural Guide. Boston: Little, Brown, 1989;245–254.
385. Busoni P, Sarti A. Sacral intervertebral block. Anesthesiology 1987;67:993–995.
386. Kumagai M, Yamashita M. Sacral intervertebral approach for epidural anesthesia in infants and children. Application of "drip and tube" method. Anesth Intensive Care 1995;23:469–471.
387. Hutton P, Clutton-Brock T. The benefits and pitfalls of pulse oximetry. BMJ 1993;307:457–458.
388. Pascucci RC. Pediatric Intensive Care. In GA Gregory (ed), Pediatric Anesthesia, (3rd ed). New York: Churchill Livingstone, 1994;869.
389. Kaplan RF, Fletcher JE, Hannallah R. The ED50 of Org 9487 in infants and children. Anesthesiology 1996;85:A1059.
390. Meretoja OA, Taivainen T, Jalkanen L. Fast onset of short acting neuromuscular blocker, Org 9487, in infants and children. Br J Anaesth.1996;76:A1059.
391. Helfaer MA, Rock P. Formulary. In MC Rogers, JH Tinker, BG Covino, DE Longnecker (eds), Principles and Practice of Anesthesiology. St. Louis: Mosby–Year Book, 1993;2591.
392. Merrifield AJ, Blundell MD. Toxicity of sodium nitroprusside. Br J Anaesth 46;1974:196.
393. Jack RD. Toxicity of sodium nitroprusside. Br J Anaesth 1974;46:952.

Index